BEFORE AND AFTER

CANCER TREATMENT

BEFORE AND AFTER CANCER TREATMENT

Heal Faster, Better, Stronger

Second Edition

Julie K. Silver, MD

JOHNS HOPKINS UNIVERSITY PRESS
Baltimore

Note to the reader: This book is not meant to substitute for medical care, and treatment should not be based solely on its contents. Instead, treatment must be developed in a dialogue between the individual and his or her physician. Our book has been written to help with that dialogue.

Drug dosage: The author and publisher have made reasonable efforts to determine that the selection of drugs discussed in this text conform to the practices of the general medical community. The medications described do not necessarily have specific approval by the U.S. Food and Drug Administration to treat the diseases for which they are recommended. In view of ongoing research, changes in governmental regulation, and the constant flow of information relating to drug therapy and drug reactions, the reader is urged to check the package insert of each drug for any change in indications and dosage and for warnings and precautions. This is particularly important when the recommended agent is a new or infrequently used drug.

In order to protect the privacy of patients whose stories are told in this book, the author has changed their names and identifying characteristics.

© 2006, 2015 Johns Hopkins University Press
All rights reserved. Published 2015. First edition published 2006 as
After Cancer Treatment: Heal Faster, Better, Stronger.
Printed in the United States of America on acid-free paper
2 4 6 8 9 7 5 3 1

Johns Hopkins University Press
2715 North Charles Street
Baltimore, Maryland 21218-4363
www.press.jhu.edu

Library of Congress Cataloging-in-Publication Data

Silver, J. K. (Julie K.), 1965–
[After cancer treatment]
Before and after cancer treatment : heal faster, better, stronger /
Julie K. Silver, MD — Second edition.
pages   cm
Revision of: After cancer treatment. 2006.
Includes bibliographical references and index.
ISBN 978-1-4214-1794-3 (hardcover : alk. paper) — ISBN 978-1-4214-1777-6 (pbk. : alk. paper) — ISBN 978-1-4214-1778-3 (electronic) — ISBN 1-4214-1794-4 (hardcover : alk. paper) — ISBN 1-4214-1777-4 (pbk. : alk. paper) — ISBN 1-4214-1778-2 (electronic)
1. Cancer—Popular works. 2. Cancer—Psychological aspects.
3. Cancer—Patients—Rehabilitation. 4. Self-care, Health. I. Title.
RC263.S489 2015
616.99'4—dc23   2014049512

A catalog record for this book is available from the British Library.

Special discounts are available for bulk purchases of this book. For more information, please contact Special Sales at 410-516-6936 or specialsales@press.jhu.edu.

Johns Hopkins University Press uses environmentally friendly book materials, including recycled text paper that is composed of at least 30 percent post-consumer waste, whenever possible.

A cancer diagnosis throws us into turmoil and for a time can control our lives. The purpose of this book is to help you take back some control—step by step.

This book is dedicated to those who have had their lives shattered by cancer. Though it is not easy, we can pick up the pieces and strive to heal.

CONTENTS

ACKNOWLEDGMENTS

E ach time I have written a book, many people have helped in the publishing process. With this book, however, I received more than publishing assistance. My family, friends, colleagues, doctors, and other healthcare providers all facilitated my recovery and, in turn, my ability to write this book. They selflessly gave me their time, attention, and knowledge. It is impossible to overstate the value of loved ones during a cancer experience. My husband, children, mother, brother, and sister provided amazing support and nurturing. My in-laws and friends picked up the pieces of a life temporarily shattered. Neighbors tracked my treatment and provided carpooling, meals, and so much more. I am eternally grateful to them. My colleagues at work also sent meals and gifts for my children and stood by me during this difficult period. My children's teachers and the mothers of some of their classmates watched over my children at school and helped them (and me) immensely. And of course I am indebted to the doctors, nurses, and other healthcare providers whose knowledge, skill, and empathy made my recovery possible.

At Johns Hopkins University Press, Jacqueline Wehmueller is a skillful, smart, and compassionate editor. Kathy Alexander, Hilary Jacqmin, Carrie Watterson, and Courtney Bond also worked with me on this book, and I am grateful for their expertise.

Finally, I want to thank all of the cancer survivors who have inspired me with their stories of healing and triumph.

Before and After
Cancer Treatment

CHAPTER 1

GET YOUR LIFE
BACK ON TRACK

I was just diagnosed with cancer, what should I do now?" This is a question that I am asked so often by colleagues, relatives, friends, and acquaintances—people who are not my patients. There are some important next steps to take. This book is filled with practical advice that I hope will help you, and I want to get started right away. So, Table 1.1 is a list of the key things to consider if you've recently been diagnosed with cancer.

Nearly every cancer diagnosis is the beginning of a personal journey that involves many complicated conversations with healthcare professionals and challenges for both the person who has the diagnosis as well as loved ones. Ironically, unlike with most other illnesses, people are often in the best physical health before they start treatment and then over time become increasingly ill from the therapies. Because of medical advances over the past hundred years or so, our understanding of how to cure many ailments has dramatically improved. Now when people go to the doctor, the prescribed treatments usually help without causing further injury. Even surgeries, after a relatively brief recovery period, generally relieve people of pain and other serious problems. Not so with cancer. People with cancer often don't know they have dangerous cells lurking in their bodies. A lump or bump, which might go unnoticed, may be the only sign. Yet the treatment is not something they can fail to recognize. The treatments for different kinds of cancers and even for the same kind can vary dramatically, but they are often

Table 1.1. What to Do after a New Cancer Diagnosis

Twelve Things You Can Do Right Now

1. Find doctors you trust and reach out to them and other members of your healthcare team for medical advice.

2. Consider getting a second opinion. This will either confirm that you are on the right path or will give you other treatment options to consider. Either way, another opinion often helps to avoid regrets later.

3. Reach out to family and friends for emotional support and other assistance, not medical advice.

4. Ask your healthcare team about cancer prehabilitation, as it can help you to get as strong as possible—physically and emotionally—before you begin treatment.

5. Ask your healthcare team about cancer rehabilitation so that, as you go through treatment and afterward, you have access to the medical support you need to feel as well as possible.

6. Keep a written log of every phone call and appointment—include the names and contact information of everyone you speak to.

7. Gather your medical information including laboratory, imaging, and biopsy reports. Also get copies of the actual films and pathology slides to bring to your initial appointments with oncologists.

8. Cut back on alcohol. If you can eliminate alcohol, that's best.

9. Be active. Wear a pedometer and keep a log of how many steps a day you are taking. For active, healthy people the goal is at least 10,000 steps each day. You may not be up to that, so start by just wearing a pedometer and learn more about how to increase your steps in chapter 7 of this book.

10. Sleep as well as possible. If you can't sleep, talk to your doctor.

11. Read excerpts from *What Helped Get Me Through: Cancer Survivors Share Wisdom and Hope.* This is the book that I wish I had on my nightstand when I was going through treatment. I published it with the American Cancer Society after interviewing many cancer survivors about what really helped them to get through this experience. You can find it in your hospital's patient resource library, your local community library, bookstores, or Amazon.com.

12. Remember that there are more than 14 million cancer survivors in the United States, and the vast majority of them were not diagnosed at the earliest possible stage. There are excellent cancer treatments available and many reasons to maintain hope.

exhausting and painful cocktails that may include surgery, chemother-apy, and radiation. Other treatments are also used, depending on the type of cancer and what it will likely respond to.

Wilfred Sheed recounts his experience with radiation treatment for oral cancer in his book *In Love with Daylight: A Memoir of Recovery*:

> As the radiologist reads off the list of possible side-effects and after-effects, to run concurrently and forever, it's awfully hard to remember that this guy is supposed to be on your side. There he is, about to kill off thousands of your favorite cells, adding up to a large tract of the body that brought you this far, and they call this man a healer! Talk about bombing villages in or-der to liberate them; talk about napalming whole forests on suspicion. For all anyone knew, I might not even *have* cancer at this stage. But bomb we must. One can't be too careful.

In *A Season in Hell*, Marilyn French, who was diagnosed with esopha-geal cancer, writes this about physicians: "Simply to treat cancer means they must violate the primary tenet of their code: First, do no harm."

As a doctor I have treated cancer patients for many years, but it was not until I had it myself that the irony hit home—how people typically begin their treatment much stronger than they end it. It's not that I didn't recognize this when I was healthy, but the life-altering nature of the experience as I went through it left me with a much greater understanding of the physical process. For many people, it is the life-saving or life-prolonging treatment regimen, not the cancer, that takes the greatest toll on their body. Of course, cancer left unchecked would eventually cause terrible problems, and I do not mean to denigrate the treatments we currently have available. I am truly thankful to be living during a time when my life can be prolonged by these difficult treat-ments. Nevertheless, having cancer is hard. It is traumatic for many reasons, one of which is how debilitated one feels during and after the treatment period.

THE KINGDOM OF THE SICK

When I was 38 years old, I entered what the late novelist Susan Sontag labeled "the kingdom of the sick." I was diagnosed with cancer. Like many of the people who will read this book, I became very ill from the life-saving medical treatments I received. At times about the only thing I could do was lie in bed and read. So I read a lot and plotted my recovery. Of course, being a physiatrist—a doctor trained in rehabilitation medicine—I had spent thousands of hours helping others recover from injuries and illnesses, including cancer, but this was different. No longer was I comfortably sitting next to one of my patients and offering medical advice. I had switched roles: now *I* was the patient.

As a patient, my life changed dramatically. Before, I had been the busy doctor struggling to balance work and family. Now I was too sick to work and often too ill to do much for my children and husband. Being catapulted into a completely different role with no time to prepare was, to say the least, difficult.

Sometimes I didn't realize how sick I was. For example, I had chemotherapy every other week in a "dose-dense" regimen. One of my close friends told me that eight days after my chemotherapy, essentially every other Tuesday, I would call or e-mail her and "re-enter the world" for a few days. I didn't notice that I wasn't participating in relationships until she pointed it out. I was just too sick to give it much thought.

Apparently, I did a lot of just sitting around, though I thought at the time I was functioning better than I was—as I learned, the hard way, a year or so later. My husband told our then 4-year-old daughter that, since he was going on a school field trip with our middle child, I would be home for the day caring for her. Her usual response to this kind of news used to be "Great! I get to play with Mommy!" To my complete surprise, however, she became distraught and said, "Daddy, when you go on field trips, Mommy just sits around." I don't have a clear recollection of the year before, but there was a field trip then that my husband went on, and I must have been too sick to play with my daughter. In her mind, the field trip was the problem. She didn't realize that I was stronger a year later and therefore better able to interact with her.

It is not easy for me to reveal such a thing, because I take great pride in caring for my children. That I had difficulty doing so for a period of time causes me enormous distress, even today. Though I know that my children were always safe with me and despite having a large extended family who helped meet their emotional needs, still I wasn't able to be the mother that I was before my treatment.

As diseases go, there is no doubt that cancer is a tough one to have. Because cancer is such a destructive illness, it warrants using treatments that may be quite harmful to the human body. Someday the treatments we use now will be outdated. Surgeries to remove tumors will probably not be necessary. Medications that are more targeted at killing diseased cells and leaving healthy cells alone are already being used for some cancers. Over time, these drugs will improve and will replace the type of chemotherapy that is commonly used today, which was first conceived of during the World War II era, when pharmacologists Louis Goodman and Alfred Gilman studied substances closely related to mustard gas, which kills both healthy cells and cancer cells. Gentler and more effective treatments may make radiation obsolete as a treatment. Screening tests will become much more sophisticated so that, instead of trying to catch cancer in its earliest stages, we will be able to predict who is going to develop the disease before it begins. Almost certainly there will be more vaccines to prevent certain types of cancer.

But we are not living in the future; we are living now. If you are reading this book, chances are you are interested in restoring your physical health. You probably recognize that if you feel better physically, it's likely that you will also feel better emotionally. Regardless of what kind of cancer has been diagnosed and what treatments you will be having or have already had, the information put forth here will likely help you. Much of its content is about how our bodies heal, whatever the injury or insult. Woven in with these important restorative principles is information specifically about cancer and how one can heal before, during, and after undergoing treatment. You may have just been diagnosed or perhaps you are in the middle of your treatment. Of course, many people remain on some type of treatment throughout their lives. Or perhaps you are just finishing up. Even if you completed treatment months or years ago, the information in this book can help. Regardless of whether your cancer is cured or in remission or whether you are living with your illness as a chronic condition, there are steps you can take to improve your physical and emotional health.

According to Deepak Chopra, a physician who advocates for Ayurvedic and complementary medicine, "The reason why not everyone manages to take the healing process as far as it can go is that we differ drastically in our ability to mobilize it." I want to help you to take your healing process as far as it can go. Wherever you are in the cycle, you can work toward physical recovery.

Beginning to Heal

You may begin to heal even before you start treatment. *Prehabilitation* is relatively new in cancer care and involves specific assessments and interventions that are designed to help newly diagnosed cancer survivors to physically and emotionally prepare for upcoming treatments. The idea behind prehabilitation is that cancer and its treatment can cause physical impairments and lead to a reduced ability to function and enjoy life. Some of these impairments can be prevented, and others, those that are not avoidable, can at least be minimized. In addition, a new cancer diagnosis is distressing, and survivors benefit from learning specific stress-reduction techniques right from the start. Figure 1.1 shows a time line for prehabilitation. At the time that I was diagnosed, cancer prehabilitation was not typically offered to survivors. I'll explain more about prehabilitation in upcoming chapters of this book.

After I was diagnosed with cancer, I was unable to work for many months, during which time I became increasingly ill. At the end of that period, although I was delighted at the prospect of going back to work, I worried about how I would manage physically. I knew I didn't have the stamina to work the way I did before my diagnosis. While, admittedly, I fretted, I also felt optimistic because I had worked out a plan to heal faster, better, and stronger. I knew what it would take, and I knew I could do it.

One of the first things I did was to address my wardrobe. When I was off work and actively getting treatment, I had some casual clothes that I wore regularly. Because I wanted to move forward, I ceremonially gave those garments to charity and bought myself some new clothes. This, I hoped, would signify the beginning of my "after-cancer" life—a visual reminder to both my children and myself that I was healing. Next, I examined the contents of my closet as though they belonged to someone

{ Before and After Cancer Treatment }

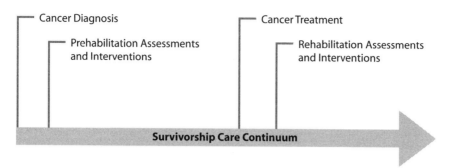

Figure 1.1

else. Whose work clothes were these? It had been months since I had worn them, and they seemed foreign to me. I literally had to dust off my shoes before I could wear them. A trip to the local department store was also necessary, as most of my makeup had congealed or dried up. After pressing the clothes I had worn to work before cancer, purchasing new casual clothes, and buying new makeup, I was ready to tackle the hard job of physically healing.

But stylish clothes and new makeup did little to hide my illness, which was still with me. I was bald and gaunt in the face with dark circles under my eyes. I had nearly constant pain from neuropathy in my hands and feet—one of the side effects I developed from chemotherapy. Any shoes except sneakers made me uncomfortable. Even if I could have worn other shoes, I couldn't walk very far—my endurance was shot. To make matters worse, I was sleeping poorly and my appetite and eating habits were out of whack. What to do?

My professional expertise in oncology rehabilitation had never involved thoroughly considering the full spectrum of postcancer care. Instead, I would deal with each problem as it arose: what doctors call a "problem-oriented approach." For example, if a woman who had a mastectomy came in with shoulder pain and a limited range of motion, I would recommend treatments that would help her with that specific problem. Another patient might be having difficulty with walking after a tumor close to his spinal cord was removed. Problem-oriented care is precisely what people need when they have musculoskeletal conditions that are not related to an underlying, more serious illness.

I realized, however, that if I was going to heal myself, I needed to employ a much more comprehensive therapeutic approach. I would have to focus on what I was eating, how I was sleeping, what types of exercise I was doing, and how I was controlling my pain. This kind of approach is the one rehabilitation specialists use for people who have been seriously injured in a car accident or who have had a stroke or a spinal-cord injury. Many cancer survivors need a similar treatment plan. If you have finished cancer treatment or if you are in the middle of treatment but want to begin to work on physically healing, then you will probably benefit from a comprehensive approach that takes into account factors such as your current level of endurance and strength, your diet, how well you are able to exercise, how much sleep you are getting, and so on.

What I am suggesting is a holistic approach to healing, one that employs the best of modern medicine and focuses on how you are able to function from day to day, with the goal of improving your quality of life. Although the point of this book is to help you to physically heal, reading it does not replace your doctor's sage advice. As you go through each chapter, consider jotting down questions you want to ask your physician—he or she knows your health needs and can offer specific advice about how you should proceed. Armed with the information provided here, you can work with your doctor on a plan that will help you to heal as quickly and completely as possible.

THE GENESIS OF THIS BOOK

When I finished my cancer treatment, I knew how to heal myself. I didn't start planning to write this book, however, until four days after I returned to work. The idea formed in my mind when the president of my hospital at the time invited me to attend a lunch in honor of several women, some of whom were cancer survivors, who were receiving awards for their various exceptional accomplishments. Hosted by the Boston radio station Magic 106.7, this annual event is truly inspiring. Radio personality Candy O'Terry is the emcee, and it is clear that she is dedicated to helping cancer survivors, in memory of her mother.

On this particular afternoon, during my first week back to work after months of grueling treatment, I sat at a table with several other cancer survivors. I was bald and frail and had endured significant difficulty making the one-hour drive to Boston. It was hard just to sit there for the two-hour lunch, and afterward I was thoroughly exhausted. But it was worth the trip, because, as I listened to one of the recipients give her acceptance speech, I knew that I wanted to write this book.

I listened to this physician and cancer survivor, and I knew that she and I had a number of things in common. We were both doctors who were diagnosed with breast cancer as young women. At a time when we were expecting to raise our children and further our careers, a life-threatening disease derailed our lives. Dr. Crivello's story is remarkable.

During her teen years, Madeline Crivello had watched her mother successfully battle breast cancer. The experience would change the course of Madeline's life, as she decided to become a healer herself. Following her graduation from medical school, she specialized in radiology. But, as sometimes happens with cancer, the family legacy came back to haunt her. On the eve of her fortieth birthday, Dr. Crivello was diagnosed with breast cancer. She, unlike her mother, was told by her oncologist right from the start that she had a terrible prognosis. As she received her award, she explained that her doctors told her she had a 5 percent chance of living another five years and a zero percent chance of surviving the next ten years.

When I saw Dr. Crivello receive her award, more than ten years had passed since her diagnosis and she was cancer-free. When she was done with treatment, though, there was still cancer in her body. The doctors had done all that they could, and when she asked them, "Now what?" they replied that there was nothing left for them to do. Unwilling to accept this verdict, she did some research and figured out what she needed to do to heal herself. As I sat there listening to her, I thought about the last conversation I had had with my oncologist, who is truly a terrific doctor. My chemotherapy was over, and I asked him, "Now what?" His response was, "You get on with your life." But how?

I wasn't anywhere close to the person I was before I started treatment. I felt as though I had aged considerably. My 3-year-old daughter would tell me, "Mama, you don't look pretty"—the only way she knew to tell me that I didn't look healthy. She was right. I didn't look pretty, and I was far from being healthy. My cancer was presumably gone, but I was still a very sick woman.

I knew that no one was going to help me to physically heal after cancer treatment. Dr. Crivello had a similar experience, and countless others have as well. Time is a great healer, but I was an impatient patient. I wanted to heal faster and I wanted to be stronger. In short, I wanted to heal *optimally*. I realized that, as a rehabilitation doctor who had spent years helping people recover from serious injuries and illnesses, I had the knowledge to do this. I planned it all out in my head, and, when I heard Dr. Crivello speak and I looked around the room at so many others who had walked in my shoes, I knew what I wanted to say when I wrote about surviving cancer and healing.

The story that Madeline Crivello told was truly remarkable, and I do not want to imply that the information I present here will help people with incurable disease find a cure. That is not what the book is about. Rather, it is about improving your physical and emotional health no matter where you are in your cancer journey. Whether you are gearing up for treatment or you are aiming to improve your strength and get your life back after you have received cancer therapies—this book is about healing as much as you possibly can. However, we do know that there are a number of actions that people can take to help prevent cancer from occurring in the first place, and we are learning more about what people can do to stop cancer from recurring once they've had it. There is quite a bit of crossover between these concepts—what works to help you heal may also help to reduce your risk of cancer in the future. Where appropriate, I will review these issues. For example, in chapter 7, "Dance, Skip, and Walk: Exercise Your Way Back to Health," I discuss how exercise may help prevent recurrence. In chapter 8, "Nourish Your Body," I explain what we know about antioxidants and whether they are helpful or harmful to people diagnosed with cancer (some of each, so be sure to read this chapter and explore healthier ways to eat). In chapter 12, "Tap into Your Spirituality," I summarize knowledge gained in the emerging scientific field of psychoneuroimmunology and the research that has been done on how spirituality and prayer affect quality of life, stress, and immune system function. While I do not want to promise anyone that reading these chapters will save his or her life, there may be tips that will help some people do just that. At the very least, if you have been diagnosed with cancer and you are in the process of reclaiming your health, this book can help you get your life back on track.

THE JOURNEY CONTINUES

Cancer survivors often function at a lower level—both physically and emotionally—than they need to. In the scientific literature, I have written about this many times, because having survivors function at the highest possible level is not only good for them and their families but also for society. For example, I wrote an editorial in the medical journal *Cancer* titled "Cancer Rehabilitation and Prehabilitation May Reduce Disability and Early Retirement." This article explains to oncologists and other healthcare professionals how cancer rehabilitation is a critical part of oncology care and will help to improve the outcomes of those diagnosed. This has a big ripple effect and in turn improves the lives of their family members as well as benefits society. Indeed, there is an enormous cost to society when working-age survivors retire early or become permanently disabled. It's good for survivors and their families to continue functioning at the highest level possible at work. Many survivors are older and have already retired, but, even if they have, it's much better for them and everyone else if they continue to be productive members of society—engaging with their families, friends, and community.

In my own work, I knew I had many opportunities to help survivors feel and heal better. With some colleagues, I developed a model for cancer rehabilitation care that has been implemented throughout the United States and is now expanding to other countries. This is called the STAR Program and stands for Survivorship Training and Rehabilitation. The STAR Program is something that institutions adopt; it involves ensuring that their staff is properly trained and up to date on the latest research in survivorship care. Healthcare professionals in STAR Programs must put the patient first—patient-centered care—and focus on empowering the survivor and family members. They must also focus on specific outcomes, including how well the patient functions and how satisfied he or she is with the care provided.

The STAR Program is widely accepted as a best-practices model, or "gold standard," for cancer rehabilitation and survivorship care. Most of the services are covered by your health insurance (not including deductibles or copays). Your hospital or cancer center may already have implemented the STAR Program—if you haven't been referred to it yet, ask your healthcare team about it. You can find out more information and also see whether there is a STAR Program near you by going on the website www.OncologyRehabPartners.com.

It is especially important for all survivors to understand is that rehabilitation is not the same as general wellness or exercise classes. Exercise is usually very good for survivors to participate in, but this doesn't mean that they should skip having experts help them with rehabilitation in favor of an exercise class. It's important to begin with getting good advice from someone who is qualified to medically address the physical problems that occur with cancer and its treatment. In Figure 1.2, you can see how rehabilitation is different from general exercise and wellness services. As you go through treatment, your oncologist and other healthcare professionals should be giving you guidance about what interventions you need and when.

It's sometimes easier to understand how Figure 1.2 works if you think about rehabilitation in the context of stroke instead of cancer. Stroke survivors are first evaluated for their physical problems and then treated by a rehabilitation team of healthcare professionals. Their care is usually overseen by a physician and covered by health insurance. When they are finished with physical, occupational, or speech therapy, they may be transitioned to a hospital-based exercise class or program. There is still some oversight by healthcare professionals but less so than in the individualized therapy sessions they were receiving. Once they're ready, they transition to a community-based or home-based exercise program. This is precisely how it should be for cancer survivors as well—they should be referred first for individualized rehabilitation services (which are different from general exercise or wellness services) so that whatever physical problems they are having can be addressed from a rehabilitation perspective.

Getting the right help is important. But cancer is a worrisome diagnosis, regardless of your prognosis. We didn't choose cancer; cancer chose us. In her autobiography, Margiad Evans writes, "Our health is a voyage: and every illness is an adventure story." This is one adventure

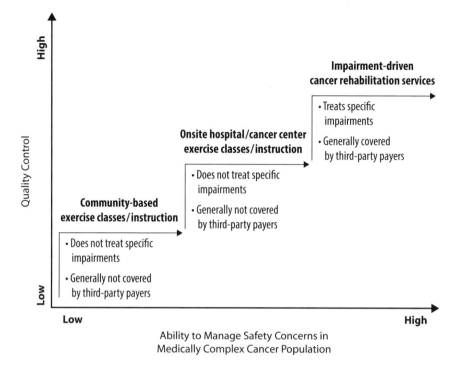

Figure 1.2 Impairment-Driven Rehabilitation in
High-Quality Cancer Care

that I would much rather have skipped, but I had no choice. Now all I can do is move forward with my life as a cancer survivor. I don't think that any of us in this ever-growing club, which initiates unwilling members, are completely fearless. I wish that I could take away any fear that you have. I wish that I could eliminate my own fears. But I know I can't. Instead, what I suggest is to use whatever fear you have as a means of motivating yourself to do the best job that you can to heal. If you have to live with demons, make them work for you. Make them part of the healing process.

By far my greatest inspiration comes from my patients and other individuals I have met through my work who have dealt with tremendous adversity—cancer as well as other serious illnesses and injuries. I have profound admiration for people whom I have watched live through some truly devastating injuries and illnesses and who seemingly handle their health challenges with grace. I have been an earnest student learning from them for years. One of these individuals is Trisha Meili, a beautiful young woman who was raped and beaten. You may have heard of Trisha—she has been called the Central Park Jogger. When I met Trisha, her outward appearance, soft voice, and ready smile give little indication of her enormous suffering. But on April 19, 1989, when she arrived in the emergency room, she had been brutally beaten. She had multiple fractures and her body temperature was 85 degrees. She was comatose and had lost so much blood that the doctors gave her scant hope of surviving. Yet she did survive, after a long recovery period. In her memoir, Trisha writes, "I built a life until I was twenty-eight, was struck down, and so had to build another. Two lives, and I'm proud of both."

As I went through my own cancer experience, the words of mythologist Joseph Campbell kept coming back to me: *We must be willing to give up the life we have planned, so as to have the life that is waiting for us.* If you have cancer, then you are probably in the process of building another life. You may have heard people say that you need to find a "new normal." I don't really like that saying—I think it's a bit of a cliché. I also think that survivors are often told to accept a new normal before they have healed optimally, and this may mean that they live with more pain, fatigue, and disability than is necessary. Wherever you are in your cancer journey and whatever the future holds for you, I hope that the information in this book will help you to be as strong as possible—both physically and emotionally.

REFERENCES

W. Sheed, *In Love with Daylight: A Memoir of Recovery* (Pleasantville, NY: Akadine Press, 1999), p. 234.

M. French, *A Season in Hell: A Memoir* (New York: Ballantine, 2000), p. 60.

S. Sontag, *Illness as Metaphor and AIDS and Its Metaphors* (New York: St. Martin's Press, 1989), p. 3.

D. Chopra, *Journey into Healing: Awakening the Wisdom within You* (New York: Three Rivers Press, 1994), p. 17.

J. K. Silver, "Cancer Rehabilitation and Prehabilitation May Reduce Disability and Early Retirement," *Cancer* 120, no.14 (July 2014): 2072–76.

M. Evans, *A Ray of Darkness* (Dallas: Riverman Press, 1952), p. 11.

T. Meili, *I Am the Central Park Jogger* (New York: Scribner, 2003), p. 3.

J. Campbell, *A Joseph Campbell Companion: Reflections on the Art of Living* (New York: HarperTrade, 1995), p. 18.

CHAPTER 2

UNDERSTAND

PHYSICAL HEALING

You can read a great deal of information about cancer on the Internet and in books, magazine articles, and newspapers. Some of this is really *mis*information—perhaps because it is old (the field of oncology is always advancing, with new studies coming out every day) or because the person who wrote it isn't really an expert. Despite the abundance of information, most people have heard very little about how to get ready physically and emotionally for upcoming treatments, stay as strong as possible during therapies, and heal as well as possible if and when the treatments end.

Historically, cancer was a topic that the media and the public didn't discuss. According to the book *Crusade*, the official history of the American Cancer Society, one of the first goals of the ACS was to help people become familiar with and accepting of the word *cancer*. ACS historian Walter Ross writes,

> If the Society would succeed, it first had to take cancer out of the closet. In 1913 the disease was not named in polite society. Patients were routinely shielded from knowing that they had a malignancy. The patient's family might be told, but they were unlikely to discuss this even with their closest friends; it was shameful to have a relative with cancer. . . . [C]ancer was not mentioned in newspaper obituaries. The standard euphemism was "a long illness." It ranked in shame with syphilis and other unmentionable afflictions.

A number of developments over time took cancer "out of the closet." The ACS was instrumental, beginning in 1913, in educating the public. But it was a slow process. For decades cancer still was not given mainstream media attention. Several individuals helped to bring about a change—including two women named Betty who were both diagnosed with breast cancer in 1974.

Betty Rollin was a young television correspondent when she had her first of two mastectomies. She wrote a book about her experiences that became a national bestseller: *First, You Cry*. More than two decades after her initial brush with cancer, in a new introduction to her book, she told readers, "When I wrote this book twenty-five years ago . . . I didn't know anyone else—any female—who had only one breast. . . . Of course I wasn't as different as I thought. But it was 1975, when no one even said the word 'cancer.' . . . [N]ot too many people said the word 'breast,' and even fewer said the two words together."

The same year that Betty Rollin was diagnosed with breast cancer, so was Betty Ford. On September 30, 1974, an NBC news correspondent told the world the president's wife had just had a mastectomy. The news reporter said, "The terror that women feel about breast cancer is not unreasonable. What is unreasonable is that women still turn their terror inward."

These two high-profile cases helped to unveil breast cancer (and other cancers). No longer was this a disease that people didn't discuss. Instead, before long the public and the media couldn't get enough information about cancer. Still, remnants of what it had meant earlier persisted, and they still persist to some degree. One reason is the long and sordid history of the term *cancer* itself. If we could describe the many different malignant conditions with other words instead, the diagnosis probably would not cause the same fear and anxiety, especially for those who live many years after their diagnosis.

But cancer is *cancer*. A singular noun that denotes more than 150 different diseases—many of which are highly curable. In its simplest form, cancer means "good cells gone bad." We can also say, more technically, that cancer is *uncontrolled cell growth*. Cells, of course, are what our bodies consist of. The way in which cancer cells defy the rules of normal cell growth and death is complicated and only partially understood. We won't delve deeply into this process, but here are some basic facts:

- Normal cells are round, and clearly defined cell membranes surround them. Cancer cells have irregular shapes and borders.
- Normal cells grow, divide, repair themselves, and die in an orderly manner. Cancer cells grow and divide in a disorderly manner that causes them to squeeze out other cells and invade neighboring and sometimes distant tissues.
- Normal cells have a nucleus with twenty-three sets of chromosomes—biological material that contains DNA. A cancer cell is likely to have a larger-than-normal nucleus and to contain an abnormal number of chromosomes.

There is a constant turnover of normal cells in our bodies. You can see this process most obviously in the skin: it dries and flakes, and new cells grow underneath what is lost. This loss of cells and their replacement with new, healthy cells occurs throughout the body. Cancer happens when *malignant* cells, out of control, continue to multiply at a fast rate and take over parts of the body. When they spread to a distant part of the body, the process is called *metastasis*.

We don't know all of the reasons that cancer begins, but we do know that for some people it has a genetic basis. So sometimes people are said to have a *tendency* toward developing the disease. Such a tendency doesn't necessarily mean that they will develop cancer, just that under certain circumstances they may. We also know that there are certain *triggers*, such as nicotine, some viruses, ultraviolet rays from the sun, and some chemicals. A person with a tendency to develop lung cancer who never smokes may not ever develop the disease. Since for many types of cancer we don't know who is genetically predisposed and what triggers may be factors in the development of a tumor, it is not possible to predict accurately who will develop cancer and who won't. It is likely that we will never be able to trace all cancers to a specific tendency or trigger or combination of the two. Instead, for many people the cause of cancer will probably be *multifactorial* (related to many factors). Scientists are learning more about tendencies and triggers all the time, and this knowledge is helping to prevent cancer and its recurrence.

In the meantime, the treatments are improving, though they still tend to be very harsh. One important way that they often work is to kill cells that are in the process of dividing. The good news is that cancer cells are very vulnerable to such treatments because they divide so quickly and easily. Chemotherapy, for instance, while damaging to all the body's cells, is especially harmful to malignant cells. The bad news is that healthy cells are injured with most types of treatment, so recovering from any kind of cancer therapy, including but not limited to surgery, chemotherapy or other drugs, radiation, and so on, can be a long and distressing process. Even newer "targeted" medications typically cause quite a few side effects.

If you were just diagnosed, are going through treatment now, or have completed all of your therapy for cancer, obtaining an understanding of how the body heals will help you regain your energy and strength more quickly and more completely.

CANCER TREATMENTS

The future of oncology treatment lies in designing drugs and other therapies that target only malignant cells and leave healthy cells alone. Targeted therapies are certainly evolving, and someday this will truly be a reality for most, if not all, cancers. Among the many types of cancer treatments currently in widespread use, however, nearly all cause adverse physical side effects. The main categories of oncology therapies are listed here, but this is not intended to be a comprehensive discussion of all of the various treatments.

Surgery. Having an operation is often the best way to cure a cancer (as long as it hasn't spread to other parts of the body). Surgery can completely remove a tumor. Sometimes surgery is done to "debulk," or partially remove, a tumor. Occasionally, surgery is all that is needed, and the healing process is relatively straightforward (for example, in early-stage kidney [renal] cancer). In other cases, the operation may be very complicated and involve a particularly sensitive part of the body such as the brain or be just one component of a complicated cancer treatment plan that includes chemotherapy, radiation therapy, or other interventions.

Surgical wounds become scars and tend to regain strength fairly quickly. Within a couple of weeks, most scars are almost healed and are strong enough to withstand the forces that come with people moving about. Usually, after surgery, doctors recommend waiting between two and six weeks before becoming very active—depending on the type and extent of the operation as well as the surgeon's preference. If surgery is followed by other cancer treatment, such as chemotherapy or radiation therapy, healing may take longer. If you have had surgery, it is a good idea to check with your doctor about when you can start returning to your normal activity level. You may receive instructions about daily activities such as household chores, lifting, or driving as well as exercise itself.

Chemotherapy. Chemotherapy literally means *chemical treatment*. It involves receiving a drug or a combination of drugs that may be given either orally or intravenously. Because the drugs travel throughout the body and affect both normal and malignant cells, they are often given in courses, with some time allowed between doses for normal cells to repair themselves. In the past many people believed that chemotherapy was given only if the prognosis was poor. Today chemotherapy is an important part of cancer treatment for many diseases from the earliest to the most advanced stages.

Targeted Therapy. Targeted therapy, which is designed to kill the cancer cells without injuring normal cells, is an exciting area of oncology research. It involves medications or other substances that are more precise than traditional chemotherapy. As with all oncology therapies, new research is being published regularly that helps oncologists and other physicians decide which treatments will work best for a certain type of cancer in a given patient. While, ideally, by targeting only the malignant cells, these drug therapies should cause few if any side effects, this area of oncology care has yet to advance to the point where the treatments offer excellent results with little risk of other problems occurring.

Immunotherapy. This category is an area of exciting research and significant progress. It represents a group of therapies composed of medications and vaccines that work in conjunction with the body's own immune system. Substances called *interferons* and *interleukins* are produced in healthy people under certain conditions. When they are used as cancer drugs, they can enhance the ability of the immune system to kill malignant cells. There is also a great deal of research on vaccines that can target certain parts of a malignant cell to prevent its growth.

Radiation Therapy. Radiation treatment uses high-energy particles to destroy cancer cells and often involves *external-beam therapy* or *brachytherapy*. With external-beam therapy, a high-energy x-ray beam is directed at a tumor site where malignant cells are rapidly dividing. Because the treatment also harms normal cells in the vicinity, it is given in "fractions" over the course of several weeks. In the days between treatments, normal cells can mend themselves or be replaced. The term *brachytherapy* means "therapy from a short distance" and is carried out by inserting radioactive materials (called isotopes) into thin tubes that are placed in or near the affected area of the body.

Getting Ready for Cancer Treatment

If you are getting ready to have surgery or other treatments, *prehabilitation interventions* may help you to get through the operation more successfully and heal quickly. I have written a lot about prehabilitation in the scientific literature—explaining to doctors and other healthcare professionals the current state of the science and how to best incorporate these interventions before oncology treatment begins. For example, prehabilitation has been shown to help some newly diagnosed lung cancer survivors improve their breathing and overall strength in order to get through their surgery easier, with fewer postoperative complications.

Prehabilitation protocols generally include exercise. General exercise such as walking or swimming may help you to become a bit stronger before surgery, but just as there are targeted medications to treat cancer, there are targeted exercises that may ward off or reduce the likelihood of having specific problems later on. For instance, in prehabilitation, head and neck cancer survivors may be prescribed swallowing exercises in an effort to help them continue to eat as well as possible during and after treatment. Similarly, men diagnosed with prostate cancer may focus on pelvic floor exercises to improve problems with urinary incontinence that may occur after surgery. Women (or men) diagnosed with breast cancer should focus on upper body strength and shoulder range of motion exercises so that they can avoid pain and "frozen shoulder" (the medical term for this is *adhesive capsulitis*) that may occur as a complication of future therapies.

Although general exercise and specific exercises that target certain muscle groups are a part of good prehabilitation protocols, the exercise should be done in conjunction with other interventions. Prehabilitation should ideally be *multimodal*, meaning that newly diagnosed survivors prepare for upcoming treatments in more than one way (*unimodal* uses only one type of intervention). Everyone who is starting cancer treatment should be taught some specific strategies to reduce stress, since it is normal to be anxious and stressed during this time. I discuss this at greater length later in this book in chapter 11, "Monitor Your Mood." In addition to using specific strategies to decrease stress, every prehabilitation protocol should include a component of *smoking cessation* for survivors who smoke cigarettes or use other tobacco products. This is because nicotine tends to impair wound healing and may increase the likelihood of having a postoperative infection—usually either a respiratory infection such as pneumonia or a surgical site wound infection. So, if you do smoke or use tobacco products, it's a good idea to stop now. Avoiding all nicotine products and smoking cessation interventions are usually covered by health insurance. Check with your doctor if you are thinking about stopping smoking right before surgery—he or she will advise you about when is the best time to quit.

Prehabilitation before surgery or other cancer therapies may also include dietary interventions such as specific protein or other vitamin or mineral supplements. It is much better to work out with your healthcare team how to best prepare your body for upcoming surgery than to just randomly take over-the-counter supplements that you think might help. Keep in mind that before you begin treatments, you will have your blood drawn, and your doctor will be able to identify certain types of supplements that might help you.

Energetics is a term that is used to describe the relationship among weight, diet, and activity level (including exercise) and the way these factors affect survivors' energy levels as well as their survival. There are many research studies ongoing about how these relationships affect one another, but it's clear that they do. If you think about it, this makes sense because they all contribute to the biochemical processes and other reactions in your body. The studies often involve looking at *biomarkers* that can be measured in blood samples. Theoretically, and as some of these studies have shown, a better diet and higher activity level correlates with changing the levels of these biomarkers, and this indicates that the cancer may not have as ideal of an environment to grow in. You can think of this as turning your body into a "hostile host"—making the environment inhospitable to cancer cells. Some of the biomarkers that may be tested in research studies include insulin, growth factors, and inflammatory cytokines that are believed to contribute to tumor growth. Researchers are studying different types of cancer and trying to figure out which ones seem to be most affected by survivors' diet and activity levels.

If each one of these factors—your weight, diet, and activity level—was a musician, it would be working in concert rather than playing as a soloist. That's really what energetics looks at—the concert effect of the various parts. For example, let's say that someone exercises every day by walking 5 miles but is also very heavy, with 100 pounds of extra weight, and eats a high-fat diet filled with junk food. Will the exercise help? Of course it will, but not nearly as much as it would if the individual also addressed weight and diet at the same time. On the other extreme is a very thin person who never exercises but does eat a healthy low-fat diet. This person, too, would be healthier and have more energy and strength by being more active.

These two examples are fairly extreme. Let's look at a newly diagnosed cancer survivor who is 15 pounds overweight and doesn't exercise very much. She decides to increase her exercise and make some positive dietary changes such as eating more fruits and vegetables. Her weight may not change, but exercising more and eating a low-fat diet will help to decrease adipose tissue (fat) and increase lean body mass (muscle). Regardless of whether she loses weight, she can improve her energetics.

Energetics likely affects some types of cancer more than others.

Currently, the research seems to show the strongest effect of energetics on decreasing the risk of cancer coming back—recurrence—in people who have been diagnosed with early-stage colorectal cancer, breast cancer, and possibly prostate cancer. This doesn't mean that it won't help people with other types or more advanced stages of cancer. There are many reasons disease begins and may advance or return. As mentioned earlier, factors may include the genetic makeup of the individual, exposure to the sun and toxic chemicals, nicotine use, and so on. Therefore, energetics may or may not play a direct role in someone's diagnosis and prognosis. However, there are many benefits of starting to heal before you undergo cancer treatments. Prehabilitation allows you to get a head start on the energetics equation and help by turning your body into a more hostile host and discouraging the growth of the malignant cells. And even if it doesn't help with the cancer, it's likely to improve your overall health and make it easier for you to tolerate the upcoming treatments and heal faster, better, and stronger. Figure 2.1 explains a bit more about how prehabilitation works.

If you are newly diagnosed, talk to your doctor about prehabilitation, but remember that usually it's not a good idea to add further delays to the start of your cancer treatment. There will be some delays no matter what, such as waiting for tests to be completed or getting a second opinion, and these delays are usually fine. But, additional delays for prehabilitation interventions are typically avoided unless the physician recommends waiting to get stronger before having surgery or starting cancer treatment.

If you have already started or even finished, don't be discouraged if you didn't receive prehabilitation. At the time that I was diagnosed, more than a decade ago, these interventions were not available. Starting early, even before cancer treatment begins, seems to help and make things easier. But, no matter when you begin, it will help. The concept of energetics and the prehabilitation interventions that I described can be helpful no matter when you start them and regardless of whether they are technically called prehabilitation (by definition, prehabilitation interventions are given during a specific period that starts around the time of diagnosis and ends prior to the start of surgery or other cancer therapy).

{ BEFORE AND AFTER CANCER TREATMENT }

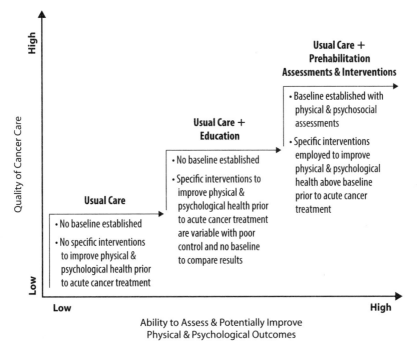

Figure 2.1 Cancer Prehabilitation

CANCER, HEALING, AND THE IMMUNE SYSTEM

The immune system consists of many types of cells carried by the blood to different parts of the body. There are neutrophils, eosinophils, monocytes, macrophages, and natural killer cells that we believe help to keep cancer cells in check. If this theory is right, then boosting one's immune system will help reduce the risk of cancer and perhaps the risk of recurrence. It is believed that at any given time there are stray malignant cells in healthy people whose immune systems are strong enough to overcome the rogue cells. Thus, these people don't develop cancer as a disease. The immune system also inactivates (neutralizes) free radicals, which are highly active oxygen molecules that contain unpaired electrons. Some scientists think that having an excessive amount of free radicals heightens a person's risk of cancer. The free radicals are neutralized by antioxidants.

Although it is not entirely clear to what extent the immune system helps to stop the development of initial and recurrent cancers, we know for sure that a strong immune system is extremely important in repairing and healing the body. Its work includes the repair and regeneration of normal cells that have been damaged by any one or a combination of cancer treatments. You probably have a distinct image in your mind of how a cut heals—that there are cells that race to the injured area to help prevent infection and heal the wound. The immune system plays a role in nearly every aspect of healing, so whatever you can do to improve your immune system will help you to heal (see Table 2.1). This is why, throughout this book, I suggest ways to boost your immune system.

How We Heal Best

Physical and emotional healing are so intertwined that they may be hard to separate into distinct entities, because the better you feel physically, the more likely you are to feel happy and productive. Physical healing is affected by many variables: the extent of the injury, whether it is ongoing, what part of the body was injured, what the health of the person was like before the injury, and so on. Therefore, physical healing is not just a matter of doing one or two simple things. Furthermore, the recovery process will occur whether you help it or not. In other words, even if you don't follow the advice provided here, your body will work to heal itself. So, why read this book? In short, healing and healing optimally are not necessarily the same. To heal optimally, you need to practice what I call "intentional healing"—helping your body out so that it can recover as much as possible. I want this book to enable you, whether you are undergoing cancer treatment or have completed it, to heal *as well as you can*. In pursuing this goal, I am going to artificially divide those factors that help people physically heal into two categories. The first category includes the three most important ways you can help yourself to physically heal:

1. Exercising regularly in a manner that builds strength and endurance
2. Eating a healthy diet that promotes healing
3. Obtaining proper rest during the day (by pacing yourself) and at night (by sleeping well)

Table 2.1. Ways to Potentially Boost Your Immune System
Regularly get enough sleep that is of good quality.
Exercise most days of the week.
Eat a diet that is low in fat and high in fruits and vegetables.
Reduce your stress level and seek treatment for depression, anxiety, or other persistent mood disturbances.
Connect with people who are loving and who enhance your life.
Develop and nourish a spiritual life, regardless of whether it's religious.

These three factors, which have a tremendous effect on physical healing (as well as emotional health), are discussed in great detail in the chapters that follow. They may seem like simple concepts, but it is essential to have a clear understanding of what it really means to eat, exercise, and rest properly. Of course, these are critical issues in every illness and injury, but this book focuses on the aspects of these subjects that are particularly important to cancer survivors.

There are other factors, too, that influence physical healing and also significantly affect your emotional health. They are also vital to recovery:

- Relieving pain
- Avoiding prolonged anxiety or depression
- Considering how spirituality affects health and healing
- Remaining connected to the world and your loved ones
- Being able to adjust to having a setback
- Maintaining hope for the future

After a cancer diagnosis it is not uncommon to feel that our illness is in control of our lives. But there is still hope. In *Healing Together*, author Lee Jampolsky sums it up this way: "To feel powerless is a common human experience because there are some things we obviously have no control over. However, often in situations where we feel such impotence, we can still empower ourselves to take positive action and choose a positive direction." Working toward physical recovery is an important goal that can help take you from *powerlessness* to *empowerment*.

This book is designed to give you the information you need to heal well, but please understand that you don't have to do everything perfectly (for example, eat an ideal diet all the time, adhere to a strict exercise regimen and never miss a workout). I think of this as the Bill Clinton "one wrong move" rule (it has nothing to do with Monica Lewinsky). I made up this rule after the March 14, 1997, incident when then President Clinton arrived at Hobe Sound for a golf excursion. While attempting to go to his guest cottage, he descended a flight of stairs and his heel caught on a step. He stumbled, and as he fell his leg snapped so loudly that others could hear it. The Bill Clinton "one wrong move" rule does not apply to physically healing from cancer and its treatment. Making one wrong move or taking one wrong step won't cause a major problem. If you fail to exercise regularly or if you have a period of depression or if you like to eat dessert or if you decide that you don't want to tap into your spiritual reservoirs, you will still be able to heal. Don't feel guilty for not following all the guidelines I set forth in these chapters. Rather think of them as just that—guidelines to help you take the necessary steps to heal as best you can.

One of my colleagues, Dr. Brian Foley, who was diagnosed with tongue cancer when he was 34 years old, gives this advice by way of example: "I would cultivate the garden of me. I would focus not exclusively on the weeds (tumor), but on nourishing and supporting the garden. I would think, connect, meditate, pray, and would renew myself. Reform my being so that I would be nourished and ready to heal."

No matter where you are in your cancer journey, now is the time to make your garden flourish, and the information in the rest of this book will help.

REFERENCES

W. S. Ross, *Crusade: The Official History of the American Cancer Society* (New York: Arbor House, 1986), p. 18.

B. Rollin, *First, You Cry* (New York: HarperCollins, 2000), pp. ix–x.

J. K. Silver and J. Baima, "Cancer Prehabilitation: An Opportunity to Decrease Treatment-Related Morbidity, Increase Cancer Treatment Options and Improve Physical and Psychological Health Outcomes," *American Journal of Physical Medicine & Rehabilitation* 92, no. 8 (August 2013): 715–27.

R. Ballard-Barbash, C. M. Friedenreich, K. S. Courneya, S. M. Siddiqi, A. McTiernan, and C. M. Alfano. "Physical activity, biomarkers, and disease outcomes in cancer survivors: A systematic review," *Journal of the National Cancer Institute* 104, no. 11 (June 6, 2012): 815–40.

J. A. Meyerhardt, J. Ma, and K. S. Courneya. "Energetics in Colorectal and Prostate Cancer," *Journal of Clinical Oncology* 28, no. 26 (September 10, 2010): 4066–73.

L. Jampolsky, *Healing Together: How to Bring Peace into Your Life and the World* (Hoboken: Wiley, 2002), p. 16.

B. S. Foley, *News from SPOHNC* 13 (2004): 4.

CHAPTER 3

DARE TO

DREAM AGAIN

The children's literature character Anne Shirley, of *Anne of Green Gables* fame, says, "I believe the nicest and sweetest days are not those on which anything very splendid or wonderful or exciting happens but just those that bring simple little pleasures, following one another softly, like pearls slipping off a string." Many people share this sentiment, but perhaps cancer survivors especially learn to appreciate each day as it comes and the simple pleasures that accompany it. If you have had cancer, you may be a person who takes one day at a time. You may be worried about your future or may not want to dwell on it. This concept of concentrating fully on the here and now is powerful and can be rewarding. It is not the ideal perspective, however, when it comes to physical healing. To optimally recover from cancer treatment, one needs to make some plans—to have goals. Although time itself is a great healer, it is not as good as having a plan that you implement.

The concept of *mindfulness*, or living in the moment, is not incompatible with thinking about the future, though. If you really want to live for today, then keep your focus on the present most of the time. Pause to look into the future only long enough to set some realistic goals that will help you to physically heal. Many people are more comfortable with the thought that many days, months, and years stretch out before them. Often people feel better when they have a sense of their destiny and a feeling of control over it. Cancer may have robbed you of the sense of future that you had before your diagnosis, but you certainly have a future, and setting goals can help with healing now and in the days to come.

MOVING BEYOND THE CRISIS PHASE

Every cancer diagnosis is the beginning of a personal and a family crisis. My crisis began October 2, 2003—not forty-eight hours into Breast Cancer Awareness Month. Actually, the story began a couple of years earlier, when I was nursing my youngest daughter. At that time I felt a thickness in my left breast and was mildly concerned. I had no family history of cancer, and at 36 I was too young to have a baseline mammogram on file (most women begin getting surveillance mammograms when they turn 40). Although I knew the odds were exceedingly low that I had cancer, I decided to get it checked out. I went to the doctor and had both a mammogram and an ultrasound, which the radiologist interpreted as normal. I couldn't shake the feeling that something wasn't right, so I went for a second opinion and had the ultrasound repeated and the mammogram read by another doctor. Again, the doctor interpreted the tests as normal. Two years later when I went back again for another check in the same spot, the cancer was obvious. I was 38 years old with no family history of any type of cancer. I didn't have any of the usual risk factors, but it didn't matter. I had the disease.

Practically everyone who has been the recipient of a cancer diagnosis can remember the shell-shocked feeling that accompanies the news. The fog of war is a well-known phenomenon; there is also the fog of cancer when you are trying to understand what is happening, why it is happening, and what to do about it. In the beginning, for many people, the words *I have cancer* play over and over in their minds—three terrifying words. As time goes on, though, the crisis dissipates. You may have lingering feelings associated with your initial reaction, but chances are that if you are reading this book, you are thinking about your future.

People who are ready to accept the next stage in this journey might have an easier time healing than people who are still in crisis mode. One survivor described the healing process as "mope, cope, and hope." Even if you are still in the crisis or "mope" stage, you will benefit from focusing on physically healing. You have been through a lot, and emotional healing may lag behind physical healing. Besides, concentrating on recovery is likely to give you an emotional boost. So, please keep reading.

Indeed, just by reading this book, you are doing something positive to help yourself. Regardless of how you feel today, you are not operating in the same manner as immediately after your initial diagnosis. Of course, some remnants of the crisis will last for a long time, perhaps forever; but in order to heal, you need to focus your energy and thoughts on how you can best recover. Brian Tracy, in his book *Goals!* writes, "Goals give you a sense of meaning and purpose. Goals give you a sense of direction. As you move toward your goals you feel happier and stronger. You feel more energized and effective. You feel more competent and confident in yourself and your abilities. Every step you take toward your goals increases your belief that you can set and achieve even bigger goals in the future."

SETBACKS

Almost everyone who is ill and on the road to recovery will have setbacks—minor bumps in the road, such as an elevation in pain with increased physical activity, or a more serious problem, such as a recurrence of cancer. When you are intent on healing and determined to put the experience behind you, you may be devastated when a setback occurs. Yet reverses are part of the recovery process. It is the rare and incredibly lucky individual whose healing progresses perfectly. What I have found helps to alleviate some of my patients' concerns is educating them about how normal it is to have setbacks and how setbacks are usually overcome with further medical intervention.

Although I believe that setting some goals will help you in your healing process, I certainly wouldn't say to anyone, "If you set goals, you can accomplish anything you want and you won't have to deal with future health problems." That is not true. Everyone, including people who have never had cancer, will have to face future health dilemmas. Those of us recovering from cancer will likely experience some minor and perhaps major setbacks. Understand this: *setbacks are normal*, they are *not your fault*, and they are *usually treatable*.

When you experience a setback, revisit your goals once you have talked to your doctor and figured out a treatment plan to help with whatever is going on. You may need to revise your goals or come up with new goals. In the rehabilitation setting, we do this all the time with patients. Rehabilitation professionals anticipate setbacks and document in patients' charts why a particular goal wasn't met and how they plan to address the situation. We know that the road to recovery is fraught with obstacles that can cause frustrating delays. Yet we are also aware that setbacks are a normal part of healing and do not mean that a person won't recover.

SETTING GOALS FOR PHYSICAL RECOVERY

Many people who seek my care have as their only goal to almost instantly feel like they used to feel before they became ill. In the first edition of this book, I told readers that this is as self-defeating as Michael Jordan saying that he would like to be 20 years old again. At that time, so few survivors were getting cancer prehabilitation and rehabilitation medical services that doctors weren't seeing nearly as much healing as we do now. Today, quite a few survivors can get back to where they were before they were diagnosed with cancer. And some become even healthier after cancer than they were before they were diagnosed. This is like saying that Michael Jordan actually can be young again. It's a pretty exciting paradigm shift to open up the possibility for some individuals to achieve better health than they had when they were told they have cancer. Because cancer prehabilitation and rehabilitation can help survivors immensely, I try to discourage people from "accepting a new normal" until they've really had the opportunity to heal as well as possible. I worry that when healthcare professionals tell survivors to accept a new normal they are underestimating the potential for improving physical and psychological health. This is problematic and may contribute to unintentionally undermining survivors' physical, emotional, functional, and sometimes financial outcomes (e.g., the ability to return to work or be employed at the level prior to diagnosis).

However, it is important to balance this optimistic look at healing with the fact that many survivors won't ever feel as good as they did before they were diagnosed—it just isn't possible to feel like they did once upon a time. I would encourage you to avoid spending a lot of effort on wishing for a time that is past. Instead, focus on today and tomorrow and what you can do now to improve your health. When people dwell on the past, they fail to recognize the possibilities that the future holds. Thus, they set few if any goals for themselves, except getting up in the morning and getting through the day. As you read this book, keep in mind that the best preparation for a better life in the future is to focus on healing as quickly and thoroughly as possible. If you are undergoing cancer treatments or have just completed them, healing may require investing a great deal of time and energy into simple tasks such as rebuilding your physical strength and endurance.

In the field of rehabilitation, we spend a fair amount of time setting goals for the people we treat. Often we set goals in conjunction with the therapists (physical, occupational, and speech) with whom we work. Increasingly, rehabilitation professionals work with oncologists and nurses (navigators and other oncology nurses) to facilitate goal setting from diagnosis onward. We emphasize goal setting for several reasons. First, we want to know as objectively as possible how a patient is progressing. Is what we are doing helping the person recover? Second, setting goals helps to motivate patients; they understand more about how healing works and what reasonable expectations are. Third, insurance companies require that we set goals and document progress before they will pay for their client to continue with treatment.

Although rehabilitation specialists spend a lot of time thinking about healing and how goals can help someone to progress, you might not have considered the matter at all. Nevertheless, setting goals is a fairly straightforward process and one that can offer you insight about how to best help yourself. (Table 3.1 summarizes the goal-setting process.)

Keep these three steps in mind when you set your goals (it's best if you work with your healthcare team, especially the rehabilitation specialists, on your goals):

Step 1

Set short- and long-term goals. Consider goals that you want to accomplish in the near future and others that will take a bit longer. The short-term goals should be things that you can accomplish over the next *six*

Table 3.1. Setting Goals

1. Clarify Goals: Decide what you want to accomplish.
2. Prioritize Goals: Decide what are the most important things you want to accomplish and in what order you will try to accomplish them.
3. Measure Progress: Decide how you will measure your progress.
4. Identify Obstacles: Consider the obstacles that might keep you from achieving your goals and address them (lack of time to exercise, etc.).
5. Enlist Support: Identify who can help you achieve your goals and decide what assistance you need.
6. Refer Back: Plan to read your goals over once a week so that you get in the habit of checking them and can make adjustments as necessary. People have much greater success in accomplishing their goals if they refer back to them regularly.
7. Be Flexible: If you don't achieve one of your goals, don't give up. Simply modify it and continue healing. The same is true if you experience a health setback. The purpose of having goals is not to feel guilty if you don't reach a certain level but rather to clarify what you want to accomplish and to keep yourself motivated on the path to recovery.

to twelve weeks, and the long-term goals should be things that you can accomplish over the next *six to twelve months.*

Step 2

Set realistic goals. Although it is possible and sometimes necessary to modify your goals as you move forward, the ideal is to begin with goals that are realistic. Michael Jordan can't go back in time and play basketball the same way he once did, but for many cancer survivors it is entirely possible to become once again as active as they were in the past, or even more active. For example, let's say that before you were diagnosed, you ran 2 miles a day. Perhaps now you aren't able to run at all, but you can walk a mile. Should your goal be to run 2 miles a day as you did in the past, or should you begin with a more realistic goal that you can accomplish over the next few months? Perhaps both would be good goals. The short-term goal could be to work up to running 1 mile on most days of the week at the three-month mark, and the long-term goal could be to run 3 miles at least four times a week by a year from now.

Step 3

Write down your goals. For most people, putting their goals on paper in a somewhat formal manner helps to give them focus and inspiration. After all, the purpose of a goal is to have a direction to follow and an expected result. If your goals are realistic and you are able to accomplish them in the near future, then that inspiration is renewed. The process of setting and achieving goals becomes the mechanism by which you can continue to heal emotionally and physically.

As you set goals for yourself, you'll need to take into account what has happened to you and where you are physically and emotionally right now. *Goals that focus too much on trying to recapture what you had in the past are not as useful as those that take into account how you are able to function right now and that are geared toward improving upon your current status.* And setting goals for yourself that are likely not achievable will just discourage you. Instead, choose goals that force you to work a bit but that you are pretty sure you can accomplish.

I have learned a great deal about setting goals not only from colleagues in my profession but also from people in the business world. Businessmen and businesswomen are terrific at developing marketing and strategic plans that are filled with specific goals. When I interviewed Jay Lipe, who is the author of *The Marketing Toolkit for Growing Business*, he suggested a mnemonic—the A-R-T of setting goals. Goals need to be

Attainable (realistic)
Responsible (someone has to be responsible for making sure the goal is accomplished—in this instance, it would be the person focusing on physical recovery)
Trackable (with a deadline)

Many of my patients are savvy in the business and finance professions, and I have learned much from them about translating business concepts into rehabilitation objectives. For example, one patient is an amazing man who lived through a paralyzing bout with polio as a child and then successfully battled both lung and prostate cancer. He has been generous in supporting the hospital where I work and has taught me by his example how to gracefully live through significant adversity. He has also given me some very practical advice on how to set goals. Thus, the following advice on goal setting is drawn from many sources, including my rehabilitation training and my contacts in the business world.

Begin by setting goals in three specific categories: (1) goals that specifically target improvement in physical health, (2) goals related to improving your emotional health, and (3) goals that focus on improving your support system. Table 3.2 suggests examples of short- and long-term goals for the three categories. As you can see, this step is fairly straightforward, especially if you don't have too many goals and they are not overly complicated. To begin to heal physically, set between ten and fourteen goals: five to seven short-term goals and five to seven long-term goals. More than that gets a bit cumbersome. In the first category (improving your physical health), set a goal for each of the three most important parts of physical healing: nutrition, exercise, and rest or sleep. Improvements in these three areas are sure to facilitate your recovery. Table 3.3 will help get you started.

Step 3 of goal setting, as I mentioned, is to write down your goals. But what if you just don't want to go through the process of writing

Table 3.2. Examples of Goals during Recovery		
	Short-Term Goals (achievable in 6–12 weeks)	*Long-Term Goals* (achievable in 6–12 months)
Physical Healing	Begin a walking program of 15 minutes daily	Consistently exercise 5 days/week for 30–60 minutes
Emotional Healing	Meditate daily for 10 minutes	Volunteer in your community once a month
Improving Support System	Ask a friend to pick up a short list of essential groceries you need once a week	Plan a weekly "date" with various friends

Table 3.3. Get Started with Your Goals

Short-Term Goals (achievable in 6–12 weeks)
 Set at least 1 short-term goal for each of the priority areas of physical
  recovery (nutrition, exercise, and sleep) (3 goals in this category).
 Set at least 1 short-term goal for improving emotional health (1 goal in
  this category).
 Set at least 1 short-term goal for improving your support system (1 goal in
  this category).
 Total short-term goals = 5

Long-Term Goals (achievable in 6–12 months)
 Set at least 1 long-term goal for each of the priority areas of physical
  recovery (nutrition, exercise, and sleep) (3 goals in this category).
 Set at least 1 long-term goal for improving emotional health (1 goal in this
  category).
 Set at least 1 long-term goal for improving your support system (1 goal in
  this category).
 Total long-term goals = 5

things down? No problem. Although committing your goals to paper does help you remember them and may help achieve them, if you don't want to write them, then you shouldn't. Instead, just take a moment and think of five goals—one short-term and one long-term goal for each category (one for each of the three areas of physical health and one each for emotional health and support system). Having something in mind will help you to reach the next step. If you are a person who likes to put your thoughts into writing, go ahead and record your goals. It will help you focus on and remember them. Also, in a few weeks or months, you can look back and see how far you have come.

FINDING THE TIME TO HEAL

One of the experiences I felt most acutely during my recovery period was being overwhelmed. Although my life had come to a near standstill during my cancer treatment, when I was finished, I resumed the roles of partner, mother, doctor, writer, friend, community volunteer, and others. It didn't happen all at once, but it happened a bit more quickly than I was ready for. I began to feel what many working parents feel—the burden of too many things to do. But whereas before I became ill I had the energy to manage the endless tasks, during my recovery I just felt that they were too much. About a year into my recovery, I was explaining to a good friend how I was feeling overwhelmed. She was surprised and remarked that it was impossible for her and others to tell that I wasn't completely "back to my old self." When you are undergoing treatment for cancer, it is usually obvious that you are ill. However, during the recovery phase, even your closest friends and relatives may not recognize that you are still healing.

If you are feeling a bit overwhelmed, the thought of creating goals and working toward them may seem more than you can handle. As a rehabilitation doctor, I have had many, many opportunities to see how powerful it is to set goals and to reach for them during the recovery phase. For this reason and because I have seen how helpful goals have been to me, I encourage you to continue reading and to follow through with setting some goals for yourself.

Over the years I have talked to thousands of people who have faced serious illness. When I ask people who are ill what they would most like to have in the world, the answer is never money. Instead, it is some variation of having more time. It can mean more time during any given day or more time in terms of years of life. Often "having more time" is combined with "having more energy." I am convinced that people who have health issues understand in a special way the value of both time and energy. Of course, time and energy are two of the most important commodities for everyone. Which is why Arnold Bennett's 1908 book *How to Live on 24 Hours a Day* became a bestseller in the United States and England. In this book Bennett described time as "the ideal democracy." He writes, "In the realm of time there is no aristocracy of wealth, and no aristocracy of intellect. Genius is never rewarded by even an extra hour a day. . . . The chief beauty about the constant supply of time is that you cannot waste it in advance. . . . The next year, the next day, the next hour are lying ready for you, as perfect, as unspoilt, as if you had never wasted a single moment in all your career."

So, before you become discouraged about adding new goals, and thus new responsibilities, to your daily routine, consider two things.

First, the process of setting goals allows you to accomplish what is important to you, because defining goals helps you decide what to concentrate on. What is most deserving of your time and attention as you go through this cancer experience? Second, you may find that setting goals gives you more rather than less time. By choosing what to focus on, you are also making decisions about what is *not* a priority in your life right now.

When I talk to patients about setting goals and refocusing their priorities, they sometimes mistakenly believe that I am able to prioritize their activities. The best way I can help people to prioritize their daily tasks is to *listen* to them. I ask them a list of questions that you may want to consider too:

What are your goals?
What do you value most in your life?
What brings you the most pleasure on a daily basis?
What would you like to be doing more of?
What do you dread?
What are you doing that is boring or difficult?
What would you like to be doing less of?

Some people are able to answer these questions easily because they have thought about them in the past. Others "just do what needs to be done" and don't spend a lot of time prioritizing what they want to do. In the next chapter I explain how to create a three-day log, which is something we encourage our patients to do so they can keep track of how their days are spent. It is helpful to write down what you do and how you do it and to make a note when you are having problems (pain, fatigue, etc.). We'll get more into this matter in chapter 4, but if you find yourself thinking that you don't have time to set goals or do anything new, then creating a log will be a helpful exercise for you. I talk about these issues a lot with my patients; below is a typical conversation that I've had with literally hundreds of people during their recovery. For this example, I have shortened the exchange. In reality when either I or one of the physical or occupational therapists at my hospital has a discussion like this with patients, we usually have the advantage of knowing how they are spending their time. This is where we use the three-day log. It is a great guide for us and for the patient.

> PATIENT: I don't have time to exercise or to eat right or to do the other things that I need to do to heal.
>
> ME: Are there things you are doing right now that aren't as important? Things you could *not* do so as to free up some time to work toward your goals?
>
> PATIENT: Everything is important. My kids and my husband count on me. They need me.
>
> ME: Well, what about the time you spend grocery shopping, cooking meals, and cleaning up afterward? Would it be possible for you to cut down on the ten hours each week that you spend on these tasks by ordering your groceries online, having the local deli deliver dinner once a week, asking your brother to cook a meal with leftovers for you once a week, and having your kids clear the table and put the dishes in the dishwasher? If you did this, you could cut down the time you spend on these tasks to about four hours. That leaves you with six hours of time that you can devote to something else, such as your recovery goals.
>
> PATIENT: Well, I suppose I could try that . . .

I use discussions like this simply to point out that the tasks we believe are essential in our lives are sometimes not as necessary as we think. In this scenario, I used a rather stereotypical mom as the patient. This patient could have been *anyone* who has been doing tasks that drain his or her time and energy. I chose this particular conversation because I have had it so many times with my female patients who spend many hours each week on "preparation" tasks when what they really want to spend time on is "participation" tasks. What I mean is that for most people, the important part of the family meal is the conversation and connection that parents make with their children, rather than the preparation of the dinner.

Most parents who are recovering from a serious illness won't lose any status in the family (an important consideration, since people who are ill can become marginalized) by ordering groceries online or having dinner brought in a couple of times each week. In this scenario, I still have the mom cooking dinner most days of the week; thus, she sends the message to her children that she is caring for them in her usual manner. Usually kids don't know or care where the groceries come from, and ordering dinner in or having a special family member bring it over is a treat, not a sign of ongoing illness.

You may be thinking, "That sounds like my life," or you may not be able to relate to this scenario. The point is not whether you can save some time by ordering your groceries online but whether you can change some of the chores that you are doing that drain your energy and use the time gained to help you reach your goals. This is where looking at both your goals and your three-day log is helpful. Comparing what you want to accomplish with what is actually taking up your time each day is a very useful exercise. By doing this, you can easily see what you can cut out of your daily tasks and add in new activities that will help you to physically and emotionally feel better. When patients tell me they are exhausted by keeping the house clean or doing the yard work, I ask whether during this period of healing it might not be a worthwhile investment to hire someone to help with these tasks. Of course, not everyone is able to afford help, but there are many organizations that volunteer to provide support services for cancer survivors and their families. Some of these are listed in the back of this book in the appendix. However, there are many other resources that are not listed. You can find out more about what is in your area by asking your healthcare team. Most hospitals and cancer centers now have a "navigation process" and many have a nurse or patient navigator. These are resources that you can tap into in order to help you sort out what is available in your area. You are probably a very independent person who doesn't like to rely on others. Most people tend to be self-sufficient and sometimes need to hear that it is okay not to do everything they have done in the past. Talk to your healthcare team, because getting help now may be the path you need to become stronger and more independent in the future.

You are the best person to evaluate where your time and energy is spent. You are also the only person who can finally decide how to spend your time and energy. In *Coach Yourself to Success*, personal coach Talane Miedaner has a chapter called "Making Time When There Isn't Any," where she advises readers, "When you can't figure out where all the money goes, it helps to do a spending log. . . . The same goes for time."

Now is when you need to refocus and prioritize. Though I am sure you still have many family obligations and perhaps work responsibilities, consider the tasks that you can put aside to give yourself the time to heal. Also consider who can help you during your recovery. It often happens that friends and loved ones are in helping mode when they know someone is going through active treatment. They may bring over dinners, help with household chores, provide rides for children, and so on. When the treatment ends, the offers of support may end too—and it may happen simply because people don't understand or know how they can continue to be helpful. Rather than being "burned out," as so many cancer survivors fear, loved ones usually are happy to go on helping if they are given some direction. For example, a partner might be willing to take on additional chores around the house so that you can exercise regularly. Or a neighbor might become an exercise partner who encourages you to keep up your routine. Supportive friends are usually delighted to find ways to lessen your burden and let you focus on healing. Remember that the stronger and healthier you are, the better you can nurture loved ones when their own crises hit.

Wherever you are in your recovery, thinking about some healing goals will almost certainly help you. As Confucius said, "A journey of a thousand leagues begins with a single step."

REFERENCES

B. Tracy, *Goals!* (San Francisco: Berrett-Koehler, 2003), pp. 13–14.

J. Lipe, *The Marketing Toolkit for Growing Businesses: Tips, Techniques, and Tools to Improve Your Marketing* (Minneapolis: Chammerson Press, 2002).

A. Bennett, *How to Live on 24 Hours a Day* (Hyattsville, MD: Shambling Gates Press, 2000), pp. 3, 16.

T. Miedaner, *Coach Yourself to Success* (Chicago: Contemporary Books, 2000), p. 83.

CHAPTER 4

{ PRIORITIZE WHAT YOU DO AND PACE YOURSELF }

T he process of recovering from any serious illness involves changing, at least for a time, what you accomplish. When you are physically challenged, you don't have the same ability to do what you usually do. It's as simple as that. Achieving your goals has a great deal to do with prioritizing activities and with pacing yourself so that you can do the things you decide are most important.

Of course everyone coming out of a serious illness would like life to immediately revert to what was normal in the past, but recovery doesn't usually work that way. Some cancer survivors will eventually heal completely, perhaps even be physically and emotionally stronger than they were before diagnosis, and over time resume all of their former activities. For others, there may always be remnants of the cancer itself or side effects of the treatment that create some limitations—essentially some level of disability. These individuals have to get used to an altered life. In the cancer literature, this is often referred to as a "new normal." I usually avoid using that phrase as it has been bandied about indiscriminately and many cancer survivors have been told to accept a new normal without ever receiving rehabilitation services that would help them to function at a higher level. Nevertheless, for some people diagnosed with cancer, the future will include an altered health status that involves physical and psychological adjustments that are frustrating but necessary.

Living with physical limitations is not unique to cancer survivors, though. People with arthritis in their knees or hips can't walk as far as they used to. Those with asthma or other respiratory problems are physically constrained by the amount of oxygen they are able to breathe. A person with chronic back pain may have difficulty sitting or standing for long periods. Hence, there is a saying in my specialty that *being able-bodied is a temporary condition*. We all face varying degrees of disability, either temporarily or permanently, as the years pass. But just as facing illness is a part of life, fortunately, so is healing.

PRIORITIZING

As a society we value productivity and accomplishments. We sleep fewer hours, work more, and spend less time with our families and on ourselves than past generations did. A busy life, even if it is chaotic and unhealthy, is something of a badge of honor. The more we do, the better we are. Or are we?

Receiving a cancer diagnosis is an opportunity to make some changes for the better in your life. We would never say cancer is a positive thing in anyone's life. However, taking the time to evaluate how you can lead a healthier life from now on is a smart move. Like most people with cancer, you may have wondered what you did in the past that contributed to developing cancer. Whether you can pinpoint a reason for your illness, all you can do now is to move forward and take charge of the matters that you *can* control.

Four times Terry Bradshaw has won the Super Bowl; he is in the Pro Football Hall of Fame as one of the all-time best quarterbacks in the game. In his book *Keep It Simple*, however, he writes about the way he questions himself the minute things start to go wrong:

> Folks, I could throw a football. But if I threw a few poor passes in a row I decided, well, I guess that old method doesn't work anymore, maybe it's time to try something new. And I would try other things. And everything I tried just got me more confused and made the situation worse. I'm sure the

same is true for many of you. . . . You've enjoyed some success in your personal life and your professional life, you've done things your way that have worked out pretty well. But as soon as you're faced with adversity you start doubting everything you know how to do.

I do not mean for you to start doubting yourself or everything you've done for your health in the past. Chances are, you've done some things very well. It's just that now is a good time to consider what you can do that will be helpful in the healing process. According to the Greek dramatist Euripides, "There is in the worst of fortunes the best of chances for a happy change." Take a moment to think about what your life was like before cancer. Did you worry more than you wanted to? Should you have exercised more often? Did you suffer from pain? Perhaps most important, did you use your energy wisely, spending most of your time on what is most meaningful to you?

When my husband was a teenager, his mother, Betty, suffered a stroke. Although she was only in her early 40s, a blood clot from a damaged heart valve traveled to her brain and cut off the blood supply. She became weak on one side of her body and disoriented, and her speech was slurred. In the span of a few moments, she was transformed from a healthy mother of eight children to a woman with a life-threatening condition. Her youngest child, Danny, was 7 years old at the time. As the paramedics rushed Betty to the hospital, Danny became a sentry on the front steps leading to his house, and he stayed there, waiting for his mother to come home. "Danny, you need to go to school," his older brothers and sisters told him. Danny wouldn't budge. No amount of cajoling would move this soldier from his post.

Betty did come home eventually, and Danny went back to school. But this experience had changed her. There was no going back to her former life. She dedicated herself to the three most important healing parameters (probably without consciously recognizing them as such): diet, exercise, and sleep. During her recovery and thereafter, she walked almost every single day. Even in the bitter cold in Massachusetts, Betty could be found walking. My husband remembers the months after her stroke when his mother would exercise before the children awakened. If he happened to rise early and she wasn't in the house, he would check the toilet bowl for the telltale tissue with the blotted pink lip-stick, the signal that his mother was out for her walk—impeccably attired. She also ate a healthy diet, got enough sleep, and focused on the things that were the most important to her—primarily her family.

When I was diagnosed with cancer, my husband reminded me of this story. He believes that the stroke, which was unquestionably devastating, changed his mother's life in some good ways and perhaps significantly prolonged her life. Today, she is a remarkably healthy woman in her late 70s who appears much younger. Her commitment over the past three decades to recovering her health has paid off. One only has to look at her family tree to know that it is not genetics that is responsible but rather hard work and persistence. When my husband brought up this story, he told me that he was expecting history to repeat itself: a relatively young woman in his life faces a life-threatening illness and responds by dedicating herself to making a priority of those things that will lead to a lifetime of better health.

No matter what type or stage of cancer you are dealing with, you can make improving your health a priority. You are already doing that by taking the time to read this book. Priorities are what we *choose* to make important in our lives. Of course, it is frustrating not to be able to do everything you used to do. But what if you made a list of just the things that are very meaningful to you? Could you do most or all of them?

Let me give you a couple of examples I often use when talking to my patients. Let's say that someone gets fatigued when walking or standing for a prolonged period—a common problem with people recovering from serious illness or injury. I'll offer a number of suggestions, and one is to sit, rather than stand, in the shower. I have heard this statement uttered in response literally hundreds of times: "I could never sit in the shower!" If you are having this thought right now, I'd like you to ask yourself whether standing in the shower is incredibly meaningful to you. Would you place it on your list of priorities? If not, then sit down and conserve your energy. There is absolutely no health benefit to standing in the shower. You don't build strength or endurance this way. Moreover, you risk falling (especially if you are ill) and use up energy that could be better used to do something on your list of priorities.

If you still aren't convinced, consider that many perfectly healthy people routinely sit in the shower. Newer homes and remodeled bath-rooms often come with a built-in shower seat. Standing in the shower is simply a habit that can be easily changed (with the right mind-set). It is one of the many things you can do to make sure that you heal quickly and well. (You might conserve energy further by showering every other day rather than daily.)

Another suggestion I make to patients is to do their grocery shop-ping online. This is a little trickier because for some people who are fine cooks, shopping at the grocery store is a priority. I am not a terrific cook, so I love quickly ordering groceries and having them delivered to my kitchen counter. I don't always get exactly what I want, but I don't really care. It is not on my priority list. Frankly, if the delivery person brings a piece of fruit that has seen better days, I just toss it out—which doesn't mean I don't consider food important. I do. My family eats a lot of fresh vegetables and fruits, most of them organic, that are cheerfully delivered within twenty-four hours of my pushing the "send" button. I have never had a patient tell me that standing in the shower is a prior-ity, but plenty of patients have said that choosing their own groceries is a priority. That is just fine. As long as you know what your priorities are, you can heal quickly and well while still doing the things that are meaningful to you. It's what is not meaningful to you that I am suggest-ing you curtail—at least for the time being. Which brings us to the next topic: pacing.

PACING

One of my favorite observations on pacing comes from Hugh Gregory Gallagher, who survived polio and struggled with its debilitating after-effects: "My muscle power and endurance are as coins in my purse: I have only so many and they will buy only so much. I must live within my means, and to do this I have to economize: what do I want to buy and how can I buy it for the least possible cost?" Regardless of where you are in the healing process, you only have so many "coins." To reach the goals that you wrote down (I hope) after reading chapter 3, you will need to use your muscle power and endurance wisely. Healing is not about pushing yourself to the limit without consideration of what tasks are important or how they will affect your body. Rather, healing well involves a thoughtful approach to setting goals and modifying your activities to achieve those goals. Although healing well does include physically challenging your body to improve strength and endurance, it also includes periods of relaxation and rest. In short, to heal well, you need to prioritize and pace.

Again, keep in mind that if you have a list of priorities and you refrain from doing what is not meaningful to you, then you will maintain a good quality of life despite any physical limitations. That is, you can probably do what you want to do as long as you avoid doing what is not very important. Thinking about it another way, here is your chance to unload all of the boring, mundane, and monotonous tasks that you never enjoyed doing anyway. The business community recognizes that over the past few years there has been a dramatic shift in what people want to do or not do, without regard to whether they are sick. As a result, many new services are designed to help people conserve energy. Ordering groceries online is just one. You can hire someone to do your yard work. You can have your dry cleaning picked up and delivered, as well as your medications. You can have prepared food delivered to your home, or you can hire a personal chef to cook meals and freeze them. The personal-chef industry is booming, and many of my patients hire a chef, even if only for a short time. There are often fees involved in these services, but they tend to be nominal. Of course, while you are budgeting to live within your energy means, you also must live within your financial means. If you can afford to hire people to provide these services, then do so as a good investment in your health.

There are other options, too. Many nonprofit organizations will help cancer survivors and their families with many of the tasks discussed above. Your local community may want to pitch in. When a woman I know was diagnosed with breast cancer, her neighbors wanted to help, so they took it upon themselves to decorate her yard with pink lights. She was surprised and a bit uncomfortable with this—feeling as though it made too much of a statement about her breast cancer. With a little direction, her neighbors likely would have been just as happy to groom her yard in a manner more pleasing to her. Now is also a good time to let friends know how they can help. You can do it in a considerate way that will not burden people you are close to. For example, ask a friend to take your clothes to the dry cleaner when he takes his own. Or inquire when your friend is next going shopping and ask whether she could pick up a short list of items for you at the same time.

The suggestions I have made thus far are just that—suggestions. For you to have a good quality of life and optimize your ability to heal, you will have to decide for yourself what tasks are most important and how you can best accomplish them.

Understanding Activity versus Exercise

Although the terms *activity* and *exercise* are often used interchangeably, in this chapter I use *activity* to mean everything that you do during the day that doesn't involve structured exercise. I am making this distinction to emphasize that activities such as walking from your car into the drugstore or doing yard work don't count as exercise. Exercise is a structured endeavor in which you work in one of three areas: flexibility, strength training, or cardiovascular or aerobic conditioning (see chapter 7 on exercise). My point here is that optimal healing involves *structured* exercise and not a series of activities that are tiring but don't improve flexibility, strength, or endurance. If you are struggling with fatigue and physical deconditioning, then you would be wise to prioritize what you do and pace yourself so you will have the energy to carry out a formal exercise program. Little spurts of activity here and there don't count— at least not very much. Running errands all day doesn't count. This type of activity does more to wear you out than to help you heal.

An Energy Inventory

Before you begin to seriously pace yourself, it is a great idea to spend three days keeping track of what you are doing. After all, one of the best ways to see how you can *save* "coins" is to first see how they are now being *spent*. In my clinic, we recommend that patients keep a three-day log of their activities. They write down all their activities and also document when they are experiencing pain or feeling particularly fatigued. The occupational therapist then reviews this log with the patient and rates the tasks with different highlighters. A yellow marker highlights the low-energy activities, a pink marker highlights activities that take a moderate amount of energy, and a green marker highlights high-energy activities.

You can color-code your own log at home; it will be interesting to see how your log "lights up." You may think that you aren't doing much but then see that you have mostly pink and green in your log. Or vice versa. The point is that this is a logical place to start. You'll get a lot of good information from this exercise if you have the patience to do it. Table 4.1 provides more specific details about how to keep a three-day log.

Pacing Basics

There are a few basic principles when it comes to pacing. These may seem obvious, but as you read them, ask yourself whether you are following them. They are good tools to use in the recovery process.

1. *Organize and plan your day ahead of time.* This costs you energy up front, but it is energy well spent. We're looking at priorities again: ask yourself, What do I want to do? Skip what isn't meaningful or makes you overly fatigued. Include the activities that will help you with your recovery and that you enjoy. If you need to do something that you know will be tiring (painting your home, doing your taxes, etc.), spread it out over several days or weeks. Better yet, ask someone else to do it for you. Try to exercise early in the day when your energy level is highest. (This won't work for everyone's schedule; exercise is important to include even if you do it later in the day.) Keep in mind that exercising right before you go to bed can contribute to poor sleep.

Table 4.1. How to Keep a Three-Day Activity Log

Step 1. Organize a notebook with space to write in for each hour of the day for three days.

Step 2. Record your activities each waking hour for the next three days.

Step 3. As you record your activities, also write down when you experience pain or fatigue.

Step 4. After your log is completed, take three highlighters of different colors and mark each hour of activity as requiring low, moderate, or high energy.

Step 5. Now analyze your log. Are your activities well balanced, or is there too much of one color? When are you feeling particularly fatigued or in pain?

---

2. *Plan and take breaks (rest periods).* A break is not necessarily a nap. I only recommend napping if you are sleeping well at night and still exhausted during the day. If you are not sleeping well at night and you nap during the day, a vicious cycle of poor sleep can result. Most people don't need to nap during the day and would do better with an earlier bedtime or a later wake-up time or both. But planning breaks during the day will give your body and your mind a needed rest. You should find time to sit down in a comfortable chair and read, listen to music, meditate, or whatever you find relaxing (for more suggestions, see Table 4.2). Depending on your energy level, stage of recovery, current treatment regimen, and work and family commitments, you may have to be

Table 4.2. Ways to Relax without Taking a Nap

Listen to music
Listen to talk radio
Listen to audio books
Listen to a relaxation tape
Meditate or pray
Watch television
Read a book or a magazine
Sit down and talk to someone in person or on the phone
Perform deep-breathing and relaxation exercises
Play a game on the computer or with a friend
Play an instrument
Play cards
Crochet, knit, sew, or do macramé or needlepoint
Engage in a craft or make jewelry
Carve wood
Make a scrapbook
Do a jigsaw or crossword puzzle
Draw or paint a picture
Write a letter, an e-mail, a journal entry, a poem, or a short story
Sit in a comfortable place with a warm drink (preferably decaffeinated and nonalcoholic)
Lie down and take time to reflect
Go for a scenic drive
Sit outside on the porch or somewhere you can enjoy nature

creative about when and how you take breaks. But do it. Put your feet up and be good to yourself.

3. *Use good body mechanics.* Poor body mechanics cause a huge energy drain. Sitting at your computer in a chair that is not supportive and without arm rests is very taxing. Standing (and bending over) while doing household chores such as cooking, folding laundry, washing the car, and gardening is also very tiring. Don't mistake activities such as these for exercise. These tasks will do practically nothing to build your strength and endurance, so you should conserve your energy while performing them, especially during the recovery phase.

4. *Perform activities in a comfortable temperature.* I know people who take great pride in waiting until a certain predetermined date to turn on their air conditioning or heat, despite the outdoor temperature. It's great to be frugal and to be conscious of the environment. But living or working in an environment that is too hot or too cold will unnecessarily sap your energy. It is also wise not to exercise in extreme heat or cold.

5. *Avoid straining or pushing yourself to the point of exhaustion.* I tell my patients to listen to the "voice" of their body. What is your body telling you? Are your legs or arms getting tired? Are you feeling more pain? Are you having trouble concentrating? These are all warning signs that you are pushing too hard. Try to heed your body's warnings right away so that you don't reach the point of severe exhaustion or pain. For more tips on pacing and energy conservation, refer to the list that appears in the box beginning on page 54.

As you focus on getting your mind and body stronger, think about what you are doing now versus what you want to accomplish. Be sure that your daily "To Do List" matches up with your health goals. Now is a time when you need to really prioritize and use your energy wisely.

REFERENCES

T. Bradshaw, *Keep It Simple* (New York: Simon and Schuster, 2002), p. 38.

H. G. Gallagher, "Growing Old with Polio: A Personal Perspective," in *Post-Polio Syndrome*, ed. Lauro S. Halstead and Gunnar Grimby (Philadelphia: Hanley and Belfus, 1995), pp. 215–22.

Pacing and Energy-Conservation Tips

Listed here are suggestions about how you can conserve energy and employ pacing techniques. Not all of the items will be relevant or useful to you, but I hope you'll find at least a few that will help you to spend your "coins" wisely.

Keep in mind that if you are going to start cancer treatment in the near future or are actively undergoing it or recovering from it, these adjustments may be temporary; they are designed to facilitate your ability to heal. Many are practical suggestions that can help all of us spend more time doing what we enjoy.

In General

Set your priorities and eliminate unnecessary tasks.

Plan ahead; avoid last-minute changes and rushing.

Plan activities to avoid unnecessary walking and stair climbing.

Ask for assistance when you need or want it.

Home

Ask the mail and newspaper delivery persons to deliver to your door.

Create a paper or electronic management system where you keep track of your medical appointments, pay bills, and so forth.

On a conveniently located calendar, either paper or electronic, post important dates, menus for food delivery services, and phone numbers.

Use commercial organizers to save space and improve organization.

Cooking

Sit down to prepare meals.

Keep the supplies most frequently used within easy reach.

Slide or roll heavy items toward you before lifting them.

Prepare extra food so that you will have leftovers for other meals.

Use prepared foods and mixes whenever possible.

Place refrigerated items most often used at trunk or chest level to avoid reaching and bending.

Wear an apron with pockets, and use them to carry small items.

Use a wheeled cart to move items from the refrigerator to the table or wherever else they are needed.

Use disposable plates, napkins, and eating utensils for easy cleanup.

Use wide-handled cooking pans and bowls (which require less strength to grip).

Use an electric blender or food processor for mixing and chopping.

Use an electric can opener.

Instead of using the oven (which requires a lot of bending and reaching), use a toaster oven, microwave, slow cooker, or an electric skillet.

Line baking pans with foil to avoid messy cleanup.

Use the front burners on the stove so that you won't have to reach so far.

Use a timer to avoid getting up and down to check whether the meal is done.

Soak dishes first to reduce the need to scrub.

Let dishes air-dry.

Use a dishwasher if possible.

Cleaning

If possible, hire someone to clean your home regularly or look into volunteer services that provide cleaning.

Decorate your home simply to avoid having to dust around extra items.

Use a long-handled duster.

Use a long-handled dustpan when sweeping the floor.

Use a self-propelled vacuum cleaner.

Use a squeegee mop or a long-handled sponge to wipe down the shower or bathtub.

Use a wheeled cart to take out the trash.

Don't buy economy-size cleaning products; stick with the smaller sizes that are more manageable.

Laundry

Avoid lifting containers of detergent or bleach; instead, use a cup or other measuring utensil to dispense what you need.

Use multipurpose laundry products, such as detergents with bleach, to save a step.

Do small laundry loads to avoid excessive lifting and carrying.

Use a rubber plunger for hand washables to avoid arm and hand fatigue.

Consider cleaning even hand washables in the washing machine, set on the delicate cycle.

Place a table in the laundry area from which clothes can be loaded into the washer and unloaded from the dryer.

Buy clothing that doesn't need to be ironed.

Use a high-quality, lightweight travel iron for all your ironing.

Don't iron items such as tablecloths, sheets, towels, and pajamas.

Sit down when you iron (you can iron on the kitchen table with a towel protecting the table).

Use a dry cleaning service that offers pickup and delivery.

(continued)

Yard Work

Keep your yard simple and avoid excessive gardening.

Ask a friend or volunteer organization or hire someone to mow your lawn and trim your hedges.

Ask a friend or volunteer organization or hire someone to plow your driveway and shovel your walkway in the winter.

Personal Care

Bathing

Sit down for your bath or shower (use a nonskid tub bench or shower chair).

Keep all bathing products on a shelf within easy reach.

Use shampoo with built-in conditioner to save a step.

Dressing

Sit down to dress.

Select simple clothing without a lot of buttons, snaps, or hooks.

Buy sturdy but lightweight shoes.

Wear simple shoes without laces, straps, or buckles.

Sit down and use a long-handled shoehorn to put on shoes.

Grooming

Sit down for grooming.

Lay out grooming products and makeup in the order you want to use the items.

Use an electric toothbrush.

Buy multipurpose products to save steps (for example, moisturizer with sunscreen).

Use an overhead hair dryer rather than a hand-held blow dryer.

Grocery Shopping

Order groceries electronically with your computer or phone and have them delivered.

Always use a grocery list; develop a standard shopping list so you won't need to write a new one each time.

Ask that perishables be bagged separately so that all the groceries won't have to be put away immediately.

If you are bringing your own groceries home (not having them delivered), ask for help carrying them in, take several trips, or use a wheeled cart to transport them from the car to the house.

Buy smaller cartons and packages to minimize lifting (for example, buy two quarts of milk rather than a half gallon).

Ask friends or neighbors to pick up extra items when they go shopping.

Shop consistently in a store you know well, because you can find items easily there (saving steps).

Check the supermarket directory to avoid hunting for obscure items.

Office

Sit in a chair with a firm back, lumbar support, and arm rests.

Keep papers and documents at eye level by using a copy stand or document holder.

Be sure your arms are supported when writing or keyboarding (special forearm rests, sometimes called data arms, are available commercially).

Plan your workstation so as to avoid getting up too many times or constantly needing to reach for items.

Consider using voice-activated software for your computer or phone (this works well for e-mails and text messages) rather than typing.

Leisure

Use a bookstand or copy stand when you read books or magazines.

Use a speakerphone or a telephone headset or an ear set to avoid holding the receiver.

Use a remote control to change television channels or radio stations.

Avoid low chairs.

Errands

Use an automatic garage-door opener and an automatic car starter.

Turn on cruise control when driving long distances.

Consider obtaining a handicapped parking permit if you can benefit from one.

If you are overly fatigued with walking, you can use the motorized scooters that are available in malls and other stores.

Carry personal items in a pack that attaches around your waist (a "fanny pack") to avoid arm fatigue.

If you need to carry a purse or briefcase, make it as light as possible and use a shoulder strap.

Combine errands to avoid extra trips.

Call ahead for appointments to limit wait time.

Call ahead to see whether what you are picking up is ready.

Ask friends whether they are going to some of the places you have errands. They may be able to drop off or pick up something for you.

Schedule appointments either first thing in the morning or right after lunch to avoid waiting.

(continued)

Ask the doctor's office to send prescriptions directly to the pharmacy, saving you a trip (it's a good idea to ask the doctor for a backup paper copy, too, just in case the pharmacy doesn't receive the prescription).

Travel

Make a packing list and use it whenever you travel.

Pack a small bag with just the essentials.

Buy travel-size items to limit what you have to pack and carry.

Use luggage with wheels and enlist the help of a porter whenever possible.

If your flight is cancelled, use your phone or go online to arrange for a new flight instead of standing in a long line at the counter.

CHAPTER 5

SEEK HELP FROM CONVENTIONAL MEDICINE

There was a time when people who were ill were worse off if they went to a medical doctor than if they suffered without any intervention. Historian James Olson was diagnosed in 1981 with epithelioid sarcoma in his left arm; after two recurrences, he underwent amputation of his arm. Olson recently wrote, "Until the twentieth century, only the finest of lines separated doctors from quacks and science from superstition. Patients were more likely to die from medical treatment than from the disease. It was not until 1910 in the United States that, as one historian has written, 'a random patient, with a random disease, consulting a doctor chosen at random, had a better than fifty percent chance of profiting from the encounter.'"

A great deal has changed in the intervening years. Today, the greatest benefit to most people who are ill is the health remedies prescribed by physicians trained in conventional medicine—also called mainstream medicine. This is not to say that there aren't benefits to be found in complementary and alternative medicine (often called CAM for short) or that there aren't plenty of treatments currently espoused by nonconventional healers that will someday be proven to be effective. It is also not to say that some currently used conventional treatments won't eventually fall out of favor. Rather, what I mean is that by far your best chance of healing comes from what we have learned in the past century from scientists who have studied diseases and treatments in a manner and assessed which treatments will have the greatest benefit with the least risk for a person with a given illness.

CONVENTIONAL VERSUS NONCONVENTIONAL MEDICINE

To make educated choices about treatment options, it is helpful to understand what it means when a treatment is considered to be *conventional* (also called *mainstream*) medicine versus complementary or alternative medicine. (Chapter 6 more fully explores nonconventional therapies.) Conventional medicine is based on research that has demonstrated, usually in more than one study conducted in different geographic regions by different scientists, that a particular treatment is beneficial. The process is arduous, requiring a great deal of peer review from the medical and scientific community, for a treatment (whether it is a drug or a surgery or some other intervention) to be approved and accepted by medical doctors. In the United States, the Food and Drug Administration (FDA), a government agency, plays a significant role in the approval of new medications. This thorough process does not mean that the treatment has no side effects or risks. Rather, it shows that the remedy's potential to help is greater than its potential harmful effects.

You may be familiar with cancer clinical trials, which are currently the best way we have of proving whether a given treatment is effective. Clinical trials are performed under federal regulation and governed by strict protocols, including the approval of a hospital's Institutional Review Board. Patients who participate in clinical trials are told of the anticipated risks and benefits of the study, and they must sign a detailed consent form. Clinical trials are divided into three phases. In phase 1 trials, a new drug, combination of drugs, or other treatment is tested for the first time in humans. The primary goals of a phase 1 trial are to determine a safe dose of a particular treatment and to identify side effects. This phase is the most experimental one, and the trials usually involve a small number of patients (that is, about ten people). Phase 2 trials involve more patients and are designed to learn more about the drug's effectiveness and side effects. Phase 3 trials concentrate on studying treatments that have successfully passed through the first two phases and are considered to be at least as safe and effective as the current standard treatments. In these trials, the goal is to determine whether the new treatment is more effective than the current standard. Cancer patients are not given placebos (inert or innocuous substances such as "sugar pills" with no healing effect) in phase 3 trials but are randomly assigned to either a group that receives the standard treatment or a group that is given a new treatment. Phase 4 trials are performed after the treatment is on the market to further investigate the drug and learn about the long-term benefits and side effects.

You can learn more about enrolling in a clinical trial by going to this website: ClinicalTrials.gov. The website is sponsored by the National Institutes of Health (NIH) and is regularly updated, so it lists current cancer studies that you might be able to enroll in. Of course, you should talk to your doctor about anything that you find online.

In spite of the rigorous process of bringing new treatments to cancer patients and all of the scientific oversight, conventional medicine does not always run smoothly. Vigorous testing methods employed in conventional medicine help to ensure that the vast majority of treatments medical doctors prescribe are more helpful than harmful. These therapies, called "evidence-based" medicine, come from scientifically established best practices. Nonetheless, one advocate of evidence-based medicine, Canadian scientist Brian Haynes, cautions, "The advance of knowledge is incremental, with many false steps, and with breakthroughs few and far between, so that only a very tiny fraction of the reports in the medical literature signal new knowledge that is both adequately tested and important enough for practitioners to depend upon and apply."

Even published studies that have been subjected to rigorous scientifically applied measures and protocols often come under attack. For example, a number of years ago, I was talking to a group of primary care physicians about the benefits of exercise for women who had been through treatment for breast cancer. In particular, I mentioned an early study that was conducted by my colleagues at Harvard, led by Dr. Michelle Holmes, in which nearly three thousand women were studied for a period of sixteen years. In this study the women who exercised regularly had a markedly reduced risk of breast cancer recurrence. One doctor in the group I was talking to challenged the findings in the study and said it was a bad idea to tell breast cancer survivors about it because exercise had not been absolutely proven to reduce the risk of cancer recurrence. Which was true. This study was very suggestive of a positive link but did not absolutely prove that exercise can reduce the risk of breast cancer recurrence (new research has found that this early study has merit and that exercise may help prevent breast cancer from coming back in some women, an issue that I discuss in more detail in chapter 7). Moreover, he maintained that we shouldn't be telling women about the possible benefit of exercise because if they don't exercise and the cancer comes back, then they will feel guilty. You may be having difficulty following his logic. Frankly, so did I. But his point was that until we know absolutely for sure—even if it takes decades to prove—we shouldn't tell patients about the preliminary findings.

This doctor is an excellent practitioner who is well regarded by his patients and his colleagues. Though I respectfully disagreed with him on the issue of what we should be telling breast cancer survivors about exercise and the risk of recurrence, I know that there are others (I hope they are in the minority) who share his view. One of his colleagues, troubled by this exchange, sent me a letter and told me how helpful he thought exercise could be—for a variety of reasons including to assist with physical healing and possibly reduce the risk of recurrence—for women with a history of breast cancer. He also said he was going to encourage the women in his practice with this diagnosis to exercise regularly.

We know that conventional medicine is not a perfect science, but it is by far the best system we have to figure out which treatments will provide the most benefit and the least risk. Nonconventional approaches vary from *tested* therapies in this very respect. The National Center for Complementary and Alternative Medicine (NCCAM), a government agency that is part of the prestigious National Institutes of Health, has defined complementary and alternative treatments this way:

CAM is a group of diverse medical and health care systems, practices, and products that are not presently considered to be part of conventional medicine. *Complementary medicine* is used together with conventional medicine, and *alternative medicine* is used in place of conventional medicine. *Integrative medicine* combines conventional and CAM treatments for which there is evidence of safety and effectiveness. While scientific evidence exists regarding some CAM therapies, for most there are key questions that are yet to be answered through well-designed scientific studies—questions such as whether these therapies are safe and whether they work for the diseases or medical conditions for which they are used.

The inherent problem with CAM treatments is that, for the most part, we don't know how much good they will do, nor do we fully understand the risks involved. The reason for establishing the NCCAM is that some of these nonconventional treatments will almost certainly be proven to be helpful. In chapter 6, I explain more about CAM therapies and how they can help cancer survivors to heal. I hope you will recognize, however, that *conventional medicine is based on rigorous research that has demonstrated by reproducible testing results that the treatments approved show clear benefit to patients and minimize risks and side effects.*

CONVENTIONAL MEDICINE: AN IMPERFECT SYSTEM

Although prescription medications undergo much study before they come to the market, medical doctors sometimes try other treatments and procedures that have not been rigorously tested. An example occurred during the 2004 American League Championship Series. When pitcher Curt Schilling injured his right ankle, the Boston Red Sox's general manager vowed to explore "every medical technique under the sun to try to get his tendon stabilized." According to the *Boston Globe,* here's what happened next:

> Enter Sox medical director Bill Morgan, who recommended a novel approach in concert with the team's training staff. Why not suture the skin around the dislocated tendon down to the deep tissue and effectively create an artificial sheath that would seal the tendon in place? . . . The only problem was, Morgan had never performed such a procedure and was unaware of anyone who had conducted one whom he could consult. So he did what many doctors do to test new medical techniques: He experimented on human cadaver legs. . . . The makeshift procedure worked. . . . And so

another chapter in the storied history of the Red Sox was written, with comeback heroics on the diamond—and a brilliant flash of medical improvisation behind the scenes that made it possible.

The Red Sox went on to win the World Series in 2004—for the first time since 1918.

I realize that some readers will readily embrace the concepts held by conventional medicine practitioners—medical doctors and other healthcare providers such as nurses, physical therapists, and psychologists. Others, who have been disenfranchised for a variety of reasons, may have more negative feelings—perhaps because conventional medicine has not given them viable treatment options or because they feel uncared for in a system that at times can be coldly calculating rather than warmly nurturing. Most medical professionals, although not perfect, are genuinely dedicated and caring. Over the years, however, I have seen doctors who don't fit this caring mold, and thus I am not surprised that some people lack confidence in conventional healers. When patients perceive a lack of concern on the part of their doctors, whether caused by time constraints, personality issues, or other factors, it can make them question the validity of the treatment. Seeking out a more nurturing environment is a primary reason many people go to alternative healthcare practitioners. For example, nonconventional healers help to inspire confidence in their patients by spending a lot of time with them. It is well documented that the average duration of an office visit with an alternative medicine provider is often double or triple the time allotted by a conventional doctor.

While it is true that conventional medicine is much faster paced, it is widely known that some of the most compassionate doctors and nurses go into the field of oncology. Many cancer survivors report fabulous experiences with their healthcare team.

SURVIVORSHIP AS A DISTINCT COMPONENT OF CANCER CARE

At the time the first edition of this book was published, healthcare professionals began to turn their attention to the problems that survivors may confront as a result of their cancer or its treatment. Over the past decade, the resources dedicated to high-quality survivorship care have increased exponentially, and more and more researchers and clinicians are focusing their efforts on helping survivors to deal with many of the problems that they may encounter following a cancer diagnosis.

An important turning point in survivorship care happened when a report was released in 2005 by the Institute of Medicine titled "From Cancer Patient to Cancer Survivor: Lost in Transition." This report documented the many issues that survivors are confronted with and established the need for more and better survivorship services—what doctors often call "gaps in care." Recommendations from this report included ways to better coordinate care to help prevent future problems such as heart disease, another cancer, or long-term side effects. Regardless of whether they can be prevented, a more concerted effort is needed to identify and address them as early as possible. Since this report was released, there has been a great deal of attention focused on how best to help survivors with a myriad of problems that may include long-term side effects from treatment, pain, disability, anxiety, depression, financial problems, genetic counselling, fertility preservation, and so on.

This report is where the idea behind "survivorship care plans" first took hold as a way to help patients and their providers such as primary care physicians understand what care they have received to date and what follow-up care, including screening tests, they should get in the future. Of course, survivorship care plans are simply documents—paper or electronic—that provide the written translation for the services that someone received or should obtain in the future. You likely will be offered a survivorship care plan sometime during or shortly after your treatment. If not, then ask about how you can obtain one that documents your care. Of course, it is not the plan itself but rather the medical services that help people the most.

In 2007, another important Institute of Medicine report was released that focused on the psychosocial issues survivors face. This report was titled "Cancer Care for the Whole Patient: Meeting Psychosocial Needs." Interestingly, the report found that in general plenty of psychosocial services were available but that clinicians were not doing a particularly good job of figuring out which patients needed these services. Therefore, this report set the stage to begin "distress" screening as a way to better identify which individuals may be struggling with problems that are causing them significant distress such as financial concerns, relationship issues, social isolation, or employment-related or psychological problems. This report also generated intense interest in the topic of distress in cancer survivors, which led to many research studies. As I've followed the research, it has shown, not surprisingly, that the leading or at least a leading cause of distress in cancer survivors is physical disability and problems functioning in the way that they did before they were diagnosed. As I've pointed out throughout this book, physical and emotional health go hand in hand—it's harder to feel optimistic and happy or at least peaceful if you are physically struggling. Evaluating this research has led me to write extensively about the need for what I call "dual screening"—looking at not only distress but also physical impairments that may be addressed with cancer rehabilitation interventions. Figure 5.1 explains more about how dual screening improves survivorship care.

Another important Institute of Medicine report came out in 2013, titled "High-Quality Cancer Care." This report has significantly changed the way that doctors and other healthcare professionals talk and think about oncology care. If you have been diagnosed with cancer, then of course you want high-quality care. Your doctors want to give you high-quality care, and your health insurance has a vested interest in ensuring that you receive high-quality care. But what does high-quality care really mean? This report identified several of the key components of high-quality care. Perhaps the most important is that the care should be focused on the individual patient—what is often called "patient-centered" care.

CHOOSING THE RIGHT TREATMENT FOR YOU

Suzanne Somers, the actress perhaps best known for her role as the stereotypical dumb blond on the sitcom *Three's Company*, made tabloid news for weeks when she was diagnosed with breast cancer and opted out of some of the treatments that her doctors recommended. She writes of her decision to continue hormonal therapy against her doctors' advice: "I'm going to continue to take my hormones, I am not going to take chemotherapy, I am going to have six weeks of radiation,

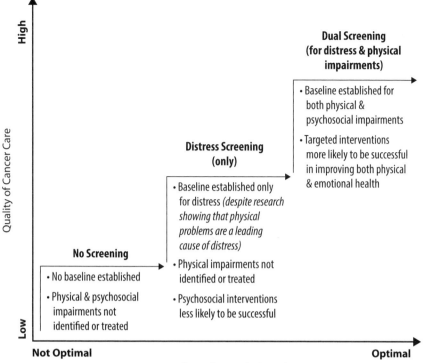

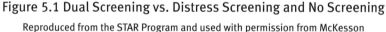

Survivors' Physical & Psychological Health

Figure 5.1 Dual Screening vs. Distress Screening and No Screening

and I am not going to take Tamoxifen." Later she explains, "Don't think I disregard traditional Conventional medicine. I am the first one in line for Conventional medicine when it is warranted. I would not have wanted to go through my cancer without my wonderful doctors."

I encourage all cancer survivors to do what I did myself and what I tell my patients and my loved ones to do: first and foremost seek treatment with medical doctors, including a primary care physician and an oncologist, who will provide the most up-to-date information on the particular condition. At the end of this book is a list of resources that can be helpful in finding the right care. A medical doctor who specializes in rehabilitation medicine (a physiatrist) can also be a wonderful resource during the recovery period (see Table 5.1 for more information about this medical specialty). I respect the right of people to choose the kind of care they want to pursue, but I hope you will become as educated as possible about the options. If you don't feel comfortable with your doctor, for whatever reason, get a second or perhaps a third opinion. Find conventional healers you can trust—they are out there.

The treatments I recommend throughout the remainder of this book are designed to empower you and are generally based on scientific evidence. Where there is not good research to support a specific intervention, I point this out and explain what is known about the intervention. Some of my suggestions will help to reduce fatigue and pain and to rebuild strength and increase endurance. They will aid in getting a restful night's sleep and in decreasing symptoms of stress, depression, and

---

Table 5.1. Physiatrists

The specialty of physiatry took shape during the first half of the twentieth century when two major events occurred simultaneously: the polio epidemics and injuries to soldiers fighting in World War II. There was a tremendous need to rehabilitate the more than six hundred thousand injured military personnel. At that time, a call was issued for doctors who would undergo specialized training in rehabilitation methods. The specialty of physiatry originated in these events and had some of its roots in patriotism and a deep commitment to helping people who have been through a serious illness or injury. Physiatrists make up a relatively small group of doctors (about eight thousand in the United States).

At first, physiatrists were called "physical therapy doctors" because they knew so much about exercise. However, this led to confusion about whether they were actually medical doctors (they are). So the term has long been discarded. Like other doctors, physiatrists complete four years of medical school; then they also receive four years of specialty training in physical medicine and rehabilitation. They are experts in helping people recover from serious injuries and illnesses and are involved in every aspect of this process, including diagnosing physical impairments, prescribing medications to help with pain, performing injections, and recommending therapeutic exercise and modalities such as electrical stimulation. To find a physiatrist, ask your doctor for a referral or contact the American Academy of Physical Medicine and Rehabilitation (information about this resource is in the appendix).

{ BEFORE AND AFTER CANCER TREATMENT }

anxiety if these are present. Wherever you are on the cancer spectrum in terms of diagnosis, treatment, and recovery, I hope that you will embrace as your first choice the remedies that have been proven to be effective in healing.

References

J. S. Olson, *Bathsheba's Breast: Women, Cancer, and History* (Baltimore: Johns Hopkins University Press, 2002), pp. 83, 146–47.

R. B. Haynes, "What Kind of Evidence Is It That Evidence-Based Medicine Advocates Want Health Care Providers and Consumers to Pay Attention To?" *BMC Health Services Research* 2, no. 1 (2002): 4.

M. D. Holmes et al., "Physical Activity and Survival after Breast Cancer Diagnosis," *Journal of the American Medical Association* 293 (2005): 2479–86.

B. Hohler et al., "Morgan Magic—Team Doctor Works Wonders for Schilling," *Boston Globe*, October 21, 2004, p. C8.

National Center for Complementary and Alternative Medicine, "The Use of Complementary and Alternative Medicine in the United States," December 2008, www.nccam.nih.gov/news/camstats/2007/camsurvey_fs1 .htm.

M. Hewitt, S. Greenfield, and E. Stovall, eds. *From Cancer Patient to Cancer Survivor: Lost in Transition* (Washington, DC: National Academies Press, 2005).

Cancer Care for the Whole Patient: Meeting Psychosocial Health Needs, Institute of Medicine (Washington, DC: National Academies Press, 2007).

Delivering High-Quality Cancer Care: Charting a New Course for a System in Crisis, Institute of Medicine (Washington, DC. The National Academies Press, 2013).

S. Somers, *The Sexy Years* (New York: Crown, 2004), pp. 22, 32.

CHAPTER 6

EXPLORE EASTERN AND OTHER MEDICAL SYSTEMS

I n this chapter, we'll explore complementary therapies that generally fall into the category of *integrative oncology*. Integrative oncology combines conventional and complementary and alternative treatments for which there is evidence of safety and effectiveness. Before going any further, to recall the definition from Chapter 5, *complementary* therapies are used *in conjunction with* conventional medicine while *alternative* treatments are used *instead of* conventional medicine. In oncology, it is really important to treat cancer and other problems related to it with treatments that research supports.

I advise cancer survivors who are inclined to explore nonconventional therapies to do so *in addition to* rather than *instead of* conventional medicine. Furthermore, in this chapter, the complementary therapies that I will highlight are focused on alleviating symptoms such as fatigue, pain, and stress. They are not useful in treating tumors or other malignancies. Alternative therapies that claim to cure cancer are not legitimate, and it's important to distinguish therapies that purport to help improve your symptoms and that you use with conventional medicine from therapies that claim to treat the cancer and are strictly alternative. The latter are dangerous, and I caution you to avoid them.

Gary Deng, MD, PhD, and Barrie Cassileth, PhD, are leading experts in this field of medicine. In a review titled "Integrative Oncology: An

Overview," Drs. Deng and Cassileth discuss nonpharmacologic therapies that address symptom control. They explain, "Known commonly as 'complementary therapies' these are evidence-based adjuncts to mainstream care that effectively control physical and emotional symptoms, enhance physical and emotional strength, and provide patients with skills enabling them to help themselves throughout and following mainstream cancer treatment." Deng and Cassileth state that integrative therapies should be rational and noninvasive: they should make sense and not harm you in any way. They should have been studied so that there is some research that supports their use in specific diagnoses. If there is no research that supports their value, then it doesn't make sense to use them. Sometimes it's hard to be rational when fighting cancer. Table 6.1 lists common reasons survivors may use alternative therapies that don't make sense to use.

Deng and Cassileth distinguish complementary therapies from alternative therapies and state that "alternative therapies typically are promoted literally as such; as actual antitumor treatments. They lack biologic plausibility and scientific evidence of safety and efficacy. Many are outright fraudulent." It is important for you to avoid fraudulent and potentially harmful alternative therapies that claim to treat the cancer itself. Instead, integrative therapies in oncology are focused on treating some of the side effects of the cancer treatment—to support your health—*not* to treat the tumor. Table 6.2 lists some of the common irrational cancer treatments that are sold to survivors and are highlighted in an article titled "Cancer Quackery: The Persistent Popularity of Useless, Irrational 'Alternative' Treatments."

UNDERSTANDING COMPLEMENTARY THERAPIES IN CANCER CARE

Acupuncture is one of the best examples of a complementary therapy that has been extensively studied and is incorporated into many cancer centers. It is prescribed by medical doctors for a number of conditions and symptoms, including musculoskeletal pain. Acupuncture has been practiced for several thousand years in China. The general theory is that there are patterns of energy flow (Chi, pronounced "chee") within the body that help to maintain good health and that disruptions in

Table 6.1. Why Cancer Survivors May Use Alternative Therapies

Even though it's not advisable for cancer survivors to turn to alternative therapies, sometimes they still do. Some of the more common reasons they may elect to use them are:

- They have a poor prognosis and are open to trying anything.
- They believe that their oncologist or medical team is withholding information or isn't knowledgeable enough to value alternative therapies. (This is a myth often supported by alternative health practitioners: "Your doctor hasn't studied this and doesn't know that it will cure your cancer.")
- They hold conspiracy theories about the pharmaceutical industry. They believe that drug companies are corrupt and don't want people to use "natural cures" because the drug industry won't profit.
- They assume the information they find on the Internet about what treatment they should use is legitimate instead of relying on their doctors.
- They believe outrageous advertisements that often use scientific jargon to convince them that a product will cure their cancer.
- They have cultural values or beliefs that support alternative medicine use instead of conventional medicine.
- They get pushed by family members or others to embrace alternative medicine or are unduly influenced by viral myths about miracle cures.
- They want to be empowered and believe that choosing alternative health treatments is the best way to do this.

these patterns lead to illness. President Richard Nixon's 1972 visit to China led to an explosion of American interest in this and other Eastern therapies.

Twenty-five years after Nixon's visit, the National Institutes of Health convened a panel of experts including physicians, scientists, and alternative medicine practitioners to review the research on acupuncture. In 1997, adhering to the panel's recommendations, the NIH released a "consensus statement" with the following conclusion:

Promising results have emerged, for example, efficacy of acupuncture in adult post-operative and chemotherapy nausea and vomiting and in post-operative dental pain. There are other situations such as addiction, stroke rehabilitation, headache, menstrual cramps, tennis elbow, fibromyalgia,

Table 6.2. Cancer Quackery and Myths

These alternative therapies are often advertised as treating cancer. None has ever been scientifically proven to treat tumors and other malignancies. Some may cause serious side effects or interfere with legitimate cancer treatments such as chemotherapy. If you are thinking about using any of these, talk to your doctor first.

Laetrile	Electrical devices
Essiac	Special diets
Entelev	Megadoses of vitamins
Shark cartilage	Other dietary supplements
Oxygen therapy	

Source: B. R. Cassileth, "Cancer Quackery: The Persistent Popularity of Useless, Irrational 'Alternative' Treatments," *Oncology* (Williston Park) 26, no. 8 (August 2012): 754–58.

myofascial pain, osteoarthritis, low back pain, carpal tunnel syndrome, and asthma for which acupuncture may be useful as an adjunct treatment or an acceptable alternative or be included in a comprehensive management program. Further research is likely to uncover additional areas where acupuncture interventions will be useful.

Findings from basic research have begun to elucidate the mechanisms of action of acupuncture, including the release of opioids and other chemicals in the brain and peripheral nervous system. Although much needs to be accomplished, the emergence of plausible mechanisms for the therapeutic effects of acupuncture is encouraging.

The introduction of acupuncture into the choice of treatment modalities readily available to the public is in its early stages. Issues of training, licensure, and reimbursement remain to be clarified. There is sufficient evidence, however, of its potential value to conventional medicine to encourage further studies.

There is sufficient evidence of acupuncture's value to expand its use into conventional medicine and to encourage further studies of its physiology and clinical value.

I am highlighting acupuncture in this chapter because although there are literally thousands of useless treatments for which people shell out billions of dollars, there are also genuine pearls that are complementary therapies. Acupuncture is one of the pearls.

Many complementary therapies embrace the concept of *holism*, the belief that the whole body is important, not just whatever part is ill. This is where the term *holistic medicine* comes from. Michael Goldstein, PhD, describes holism this way: "Some forms of CAM are not at all holistic. For example, the use of an unproved drug, such as Laetrile, is no more holistic than the use of conventional chemotherapy. . . . Holism demands a total rejection of the mind-body dualism that has characterized so much of conventional 'scientific' medicine. Instead, what is emphasized is the uniqueness of the factors that produce health or illness for each individual." Indeed, as Dr. Goldstein also notes, the key to holistic medicine is figuring out in what ways a particular patient is different from other patients who may share the same illness. The uniqueness of the patient, not the disease, guides the therapy.

Another important concept in CAM is *vitalism*, which refers to the belief that there is a life force that helps to promote health and healing. Associated with this concept is the idea that illness results from imbalance or blockage of an essential flow of energy. Restoring balance is therefore often the goal. Spirituality may be a part of CAM, though many CAM therapies utilize nonreligious forms of spirituality such as meditation and relaxation techniques. Also common to most CAM therapies is the belief that health is not just the absence of illness but a positive state. Health is a goal to be gained by effort rather than just good luck. In this view, the individual has a responsibility to achieve balance and promote wellness (for example, by meditating or following a specific diet). Conventional medicine is more concerned with the pathology of a particular illness, including its cause and effect. The emphasis is not holistic, since treatments target a particular problem. A simple example is using penicillin to treat a bacterial infection.

LEGITIMATING SOME COMPLEMENTARY THERAPIES

In 1993 Harvard physician and researcher David Eisenberg and his colleagues published a report titled "Unconventional Medicine in the United States: Prevalence, Costs, and Patterns of Use." Eisenberg reported that approximately one of every three Americans was using

CAM therapies and that approximately two of every three people who did so were not telling their primary health provider about it.

Following this landmark study, the NIH established the Office for the Study of Unconventional Medical Practices. The creation of this office was the beginning of the attempt to legitimate CAM therapies that are truly beneficial. The office has worked toward providing the foundation for rigorous testing of CAM treatments, so that we can better understand scientifically which are helpful and which are harmful—or simply useless.

Five years after the creation of the new office, Eisenberg and his colleagues published another study of CAM use. Their survey defined CAM as those interventions "neither taught widely in medical schools nor generally available in U.S. hospitals." This time they found that the percentage of Americans using CAM had risen from 33.8 percent to 42.1 percent and that the estimated out-of-pocket expenses had increased from just over $13 billion to approximately $27 billion. The same year, the NIH elevated its recently established office to the status of a center and renamed it the National Center for Complementary and Alternative Medicine (NCCAM).

The NCCAM is "the Federal Government's lead agency for scientific research on CAM. The NCCAM is dedicated to exploring complementary and alternative healing practices in the context of rigorous science, training CAM researchers, and disseminating authoritative information to the public and professionals." Stated more simply, the NCCAM is dedicated to validating those treatments and practitioners that stand up to vigorous scientific study and to driving out the mystics and charlatans who prey on people who are sick and vulnerable.

The NCCAM is also working to dispel myths about CAM treatments so that Americans can choose therapies that are likely to have some benefit and minimal risk of serious side effects. For example, a common belief among CAM users is that herbal remedies are safe because they are "natural." *This is absolutely not true.* The most worrisome example is nicotine, which was once thought to be safe because it occurs in nature. Research on another widely used natural substance, St. John's wort, reveals that it may influence the effectiveness of other prescription drugs it is taken alongside. John Horn, professor of pharmacy at the University of Washington in Seattle and coauthor of the medical handbook *The Top 100 Drug Interactions*, told me that "St. John's wort interacts with about half the drugs on the market."

A third example of how herbal treatments (which do not currently have to undergo the rigorous Food and Drug Administration approval process that prescription drugs do) might be harmful comes from research conducted by Dr. Robert Saper of Harvard Medical School and his colleagues. In one study published in the highly respected *Journal of the American Medical Association*, Saper looked at the heavy metal content of Ayurvedic herbal medicine products. The results from the study are as follows: "Lead, mercury, and arsenic intoxication have been associated with the use of Ayurvedic herbal medicine products. . . . One of 5 Ayurvedic herbal medicine products produced in South Asia and available in Boston South Asian grocery stores contains potentially harmful levels of lead, mercury, and/or arsenic. Users of Ayurvedic medicine may be at risk for heavy metal toxicity, and testing of Ayurvedic herbal medicine products for toxic heavy metals should be mandatory."

The NCCAM supported Saper's research on this topic, and I hope this information will lead to safer Ayurvedic medicine products for those who want to take them. Of course, there are also many other CAM therapy issues that the NCCAM is attempting to address. Although there is much we don't know about these treatments, I want to share with you what we do know about them with respect to healing and cancer.

TYPES OF CAM THERAPIES

It is helpful to divide CAM therapies into five categories:

1. Alternative medical systems
2. Mind-body interventions
3. Biologically based therapies
4. Manipulative and body-based methods
5. Energy therapies

Although this section is not a complete list of CAM therapies by any means, I will provide examples of each of the five categories. If you are using any of these therapies or considering trying them, please discuss this with your healthcare team.

Alternative Medical Systems

Homeopathy. Homeopathy dates back to the Greek physician Hippocrates, who established some of its basic principles in the fifth century B.C. Hippocrates believed that it was essential to understand people's symptoms and how they react to disease in order to treat them. Although understanding the whole person is a founding principle in homeopathy, the field wasn't fully established until the German physician and chemist Samuel Hahnemann (1755–1843) began experimenting on himself. Dr. Hahnemann had become disillusioned with medicine at a time disease was rampant and treatments were increasingly invasive and often brutal. Although he did not have malaria, Hahnemann tried one of the common malaria treatments of the time on himself. He began to take quinine and found that he was starting to experience the symptoms of malaria despite not having the disease. When he stopped the quinine, his symptoms disappeared.

From this experiment came others, upon which the basic principles of homeopathy were formulated: that the body is trying to heal itself and that giving someone treatments that are similar to the symptoms of the illness will help to treat the condition. This theory, "like cures like," or in Latin *similia similibus curantur*, is called the law of similars and is in contrast to *allopathic* (conventional) medicine, the mainstay of medical treatment in most developed countries.

For example, if a patient is experiencing diarrhea, an allopathic physician would typically prescribe something to harden the stool, whereas a homeopathic physician would prescribe a minute amount of something that causes diarrhea if given in larger doses. Because "homeopathic doses" are very small and usually come from "natural" substances (plants, minerals, venom of poisonous snakes, ink of the cuttlefish, and so forth), they are often promoted as being safe for everyone, including babies. Proponents of evidence-based medical approaches commonly counter this view with the fact that nicotine is a naturally occurring substance that can be harmful. This is not to imply that legitimate homeopathic doctors would prescribe nicotine, but rather that we really don't know much about any substance that has not undergone rigorous scientific inquiry. Homeopathic treatments are not subject to the same regulations as the manufacturing and sale of prescription drugs. Most homeopathic remedies are available without a prescription.

Traditional Chinese Medicine. Traditional Chinese medicine has two major components, acupuncture and herbal remedies. Although many people equate Chinese medicine with acupuncture, the use of herbs is the cornerstone of the system. But taking an herbal Chinese remedy is not the same thing as taking a prescription drug for a particular condition. Conventional medicine is concerned with how the body operates and what can be proven to help with illness. Chinese medicine is intertwined with a philosophy about life that has to do with balance and involves the concepts of *yin* and *yang*. To be a balanced person, one cannot have an over- or underexpression of either. Instead, they must be working together in balance. Chi is another important concept in traditional Chinese medicine; it can be loosely defined as the vital energy of the universe or the energy that binds yin and yang. This Chinese medical system is quite intricate, with many layers of philosophy that healers adhere to. For example, subcategories of yin and yang include cold and heat, internal and external, and deficiency and excess. When they work in harmony, you remain healthy; imbalances cause illness. For instance, too much heat in the body (for example, hot, swollen joints) indicates an excess of yang.

Ayurvedic Medicine. This ancient medical system from India and Sri Lanka is similar to traditional Chinese medicine in that it intertwines health and a philosophy of life. It is said that perhaps five thousand years ago, the great sages or seers of India discovered Veda, the knowledge of how our world works. In Sanskrit *Ayu* means "life" and *Veda* means "knowledge." Ayurveda is a complex system of healing that utilizes the fundamental belief that everything in our universe is composed of energy, or *prana*. To remain healthy, we must live in a way that encourages energy balance. There are three energies in the body, known as the three *dosa*, or the *tridosa*. The Sanskrit names for these are *vatha*, *pitha*, and *kapha*. All three dosa govern a person's constitution as well as hair color, weight gain, and so on. If kapha dominates, for instance, then you are a "kapha type." Kapha people tend to be large and rounded and are likely to overindulge in certain foods, such as hard cheeses, sugar, and fried foods. All disturbances in health are related to these three dosa. (The Ayurvedic medical system is much more complex than what is presented here.) Dr. Christine Horner, an allopathic plastic surgeon who is an advocate of the Ayurvedic medicine tradition, sums it up this way:

Although Ayurveda is thousands of years old, it is an extremely sophisticated system of medicine that has many specialty divisions—branches of medicine—that have lasted through time. . . . If you've ever looked into using complementary and alternative medicine (CAM), I'd be surprised if you didn't become confused and overwhelmed. On the surface, it appears to be a smorgasbord of hundreds of different health practices with no apparent link. . . . Most of the techniques used in CAM today have their roots in Ayurveda, including such diverse treatments as yoga, massage, meditation, music therapy, sound therapy, aromatherapy, herbs, breathing techniques, special diets, and detoxification, to name just a few.

Mind-Body Interventions

Meditation. Meditation is the ability to self-regulate your thoughts in order to suspend your normal stream of consciousness. A common goal of meditation, which distinguishes it from relaxation, is to reach a state of "thoughtless awareness" during which you are passively aware of sensations at the present moment. There are a number of different methods that people use to meditate. The methods that involve the constant repetition of sounds or images without aiming for a state of thoughtless awareness are sometimes called quasimeditative. Meditation is generally thought to be safe for most people. (Meditation is explored in more detail in chapter 12.)

Prayer. Prayer can be defined as asking for something while aiming to connect with God or some other object of worship. Prayer has been a part of healing for a *very* long time. People can pray for themselves or for others. Intercessory prayer is prayer on behalf of others. Of note is that prayer is generally believed to be safe. Praying for oneself has been shown to be beneficial in a number of studies for various health issues. Intercessory prayer is more controversial and has had conflicting research results. (Prayer as a healing aid is discussed in greater detail in chapter 12.)

Biologically Based Therapies

Botanicals, Dietary Supplements, and Herbal Products. Herbs are a subset of *botanicals*, a term meaning plants or plant parts that are valued for their medicinal properties. Any herbal or botanical products, or "phytomedicines," may be considered botanicals. In the 1994 Dietary Supplement Health and Education Act, Congress defined a dietary supplement as a product (other than tobacco) taken by mouth that contains a "dietary ingredient" that is intended to supplement the diet. Dietary ingredients may include vitamins, minerals, herbs or other botanicals, amino acids, and substances such as enzymes, organ tissues, and metabolites.

Under the act, dietary supplements are considered food, not drugs, and therefore are not subject to FDA oversight. Before marketing a prescription drug, manufacturers must provide the FDA with convincing evidence that the drug is safe and effective. Botanical manufacturers are not required to provide the FDA with convincing evidence that their product is safe and effective. However, the FDA may remove a botanical product from the market if the label is misleading.

For example, in 2015, New York's attorney general Eric Schneiderman wrote cease and desist letters to four major retailers, Target, Walmart, Walgreens, and GNC, because he alleged their store brand supplements did not contain the ingredients that were advertised on the product labels. According to Schneiderman, when products such as St. John's wort, ginseng, and echinacea were tested, only 21% of them contained the ingredients on the label. Walmart was alleged to be the biggest offender, with only 4% of its products containing the advertised ingredients. Attorney General Schneiderman stated, "This investigation makes one thing abundantly clear: the old adage 'buyer beware' may be especially true for consumers of herbal supplements." He noted that the DNA testing of the products confirmed long-standing questions about the herbal supplement industry and reminded retailers that mislabeling, contamination, and false advertising are illegal.

The action of botanicals ranges from mild to potent and depends on the plant or combination of plants used, how they were manufactured (including contaminants), and who is taking them. Just as with prescription drugs, botanicals can have any number of side effects, from annoying to life threatening. In an article titled "Complementary and Alternative Therapies for Cancer," the authors, who are part of the Integrative Medicine Service at Memorial Sloan-Kettering Cancer Center, state:

> The general public tends not to be aware that herbs are dilute natural drugs that contain scores of different chemicals, most of which have not been documented. Their effects are not always predictable. Neither the FDA nor any other agency examines herbal remedies for safety and effectiveness. Few products have been formally tested for side effects or quality control. Patients undergoing active treatment should be told to stop using herbal remedies, because some herbs cause problematic interactions with chemotherapeutic agents, sensitization of the skin to radiation therapy, dangerous blood pressure swings, and other unwanted interactions with anesthetics during surgery.

If you are taking herbs or dietary supplements or are considering taking them, talk to your oncologist and your primary care physician about possible side effects and interactions with other medications or treatments you are receiving.

Manipulative and Body-Based Methods

Osteopathic and Chiropractic Manipulation. Osteopathy was founded by a medical doctor, Andrew Taylor Still, in 1874. Dr. Still sought to develop a holistic approach to medicine that would incorporate the body's natural healing powers. Today, doctors of osteopathic medicine (DOs) are trained in a manner similar to that of medical doctors (MDs); they also receive training in "manual" medicine and manipulation. Osteopaths are able to hold the same hospital privileges as medical doctors, and they are skilled at ordering appropriate tests and prescribing drugs.

Chiropractic medicine stems from the work of David Daniel Palmer, who in the late 1800s came to believe that abnormal nerve function could cause illness. He theorized that spinal manipulation could improve a person's health. Palmer's ideas were not well received in the medical community, and some early chiropractors, including Palmer, were imprisoned. Thus began a long and often contentious relationship between conventional doctors and chiropractors. In the 1970s, the American Medical Association (which represents medical doctors) was successfully sued by chiropractors for bias in an antitrust case. Chiropractors now attend accredited colleges and have national guidelines and standards that they must adhere to. Chiropractors are not the same as osteopaths, however; they do not have the same training or privileges (for example, to prescribe medications) that medical doctors and osteopaths share.

There are some serious, though uncommon, risks associated with manipulation of the spine or other body parts. All manipulation should be done by a skilled practitioner. It is not advisable to undergo manipulation if you have osteoporosis or cancer that affects the bones. People with a history of stroke, problems with their blood vessels such as clogging of the arteries in the neck, or aneurysms should generally avoid spinal or other types of manipulation. The practice of manipulation carries inherent risks and can in rare cases lead to nerve and spinal cord injury, stroke, and bone fractures.

Therapeutic Massage. Therapeutic massage is manipulation of the soft tissues of the body and can be done using a variety of techniques, including rubbing, kneading, pressing, rolling, and slapping. Touch is central to massage, though massage therapists may use different parts of their body for various techniques (such as fingers, palms, or elbows). There are many different names for massage techniques (manual lymph drainage, Swedish massage, deep tissue massage, Rolfing, and others). Some of the techniques are gentle and others are quite forceful. Massage has been shown to help promote blood and lymphatic circulation as well as to relax muscles and relieve pain. The practice of massage dates back thousands of years and can be traced to many ancient cultures. Generally there are three primary therapeutic benefits of massage—relaxation, pain relief, and improved sleep—all of which are important in healing. There may be other benefits as well, though these are more controversial (for example, decreasing cortisol levels and improving immune response). Massage is generally thought to be safe as long as it is not overly forceful. But doctors do not usually advise having massage done over an area where you have a tumor. Also, if you are taking an anticoagulant or if you have severe osteoporosis, it may be wise to avoid massage. Your doctor may give you other precautions.

Energy Therapies

Reiki. *Reiki* is a Japanese word that comes from *rei*, meaning "universal spirit," and *ki*, meaning "life energy." Reiki is an ancient healing method that was revitalized in the 1800s by the Buddhist monk Hichau Mikao Usui. Practitioners believe that the health benefits of Reiki come from a "universal life energy" that they are able to channel to patients. Reiki masters position their hands in twelve to fifteen different places on the individual's body and hold them in each place for 2–5 minutes. They may put their hands directly on the person (who is wearing clothes) or hold their hands one to two inches above the person's flesh. Sometimes masters use a technique called "sweeping," which is passing their hands over the person to detect areas of energy disruption. There are five basic principles of Reiki:

1. Just for today, do not worry.
2. Just for today, do not anger.
3. Honor your parents, teachers, and elders.
4. Earn your living honestly.
5. Show gratitude to every living thing.

Reiki advocates believe that the treatments leave them enlightened, with improved mental clarity, well-being, and spirituality. It has been proposed that Reiki may lower heart rate and blood pressure, boost the immune system, alter hormone levels, and stimulate endorphins (the body's natural painkillers). These claims have not yet been well studied. Reiki is generally thought to be safe when practiced in the manner described above.

Therapeutic Touch. Delores Krieger, RN, PhD, and Dora Kunz, a natural healer, developed this mode of therapy in the 1970s. Although therapeutic touch has ancient origins that come from both religious and secular practices and includes healing from the "laying on" of hands, it is now most commonly used by nurses and mental health practitioners. Therapeutic touch is not meant to have religious connotations; however, there is debate in the scientific community over whether the method should be classified as a religious or spiritual approach rather than a therapeutic intervention. The basic concept is that a "life energy" imbalance can potentially be corrected with treatment. During treatment, practitioners hold their hands a short distance from a patient without making physical contact. Therapeutic touch is generally thought to be safe, since it does not involve physical contact between the patient and the practitioner; however, its effectiveness is controversial.

Cancer and CAM

Cancer patients make more use of CAM treatments than the general population does, according to a number of studies. For example, a review of twenty-one research studies found that in some reports up to 95 percent of the participants were using some form of CAM. In this same review, the researchers noted that many people did not tell their doctors that they were using CAM—in fact, in some studies, nearly 80 percent of participants didn't inform their doctors. It's very important to let your doctors know all of the medications and over-the-counter supplements that you are taking as well as any other types of healthcare interventions you are employing, including CAM. It probably is no surprise that many of us who have faced cancer are willing to try therapies outside of mainstream medicine. As one study in the book *Evidence-Based Cancer Care and Prevention* pointed out, "Cancer patients are a highly vulnerable population, often looking for a cure or relief of symptoms from nearly any source and often at whatever price is requested."

Around the issue of CAM therapies, tempers sometimes flare. I remember a conversation with a group of my colleagues and their wives. A woman who is married to a physician lamented that one of her friends, who had breast cancer, was not willing to try CAM treatments. The doctor's wife, despite her husband's occupation, had a great dislike for mainstream medicine. This dated back to experiences with her father, when she believed the conventional medical establishment had let him down. Her friend with cancer, however, had supreme faith in her doctors and did not want to try anything that was not proven to be effective. The two women, though close friends, had very different opinions about this topic. My goal here is simply to provide the most up-to-date information so that you can make decisions that are right for you. In Table 6.3, I list some potentially helpful complementary therapies and describe how they might support healing.

BEWARE THE CHARLATANS, MYSTICS, AND QUACKS

I advise people not to rely solely on nonconventional practitioners, though I believe that some of them can be very helpful. I do not want to taint legitimate alternative healers, but I want you to be aware of the booming CAM industry and to recognize its long and often sordid history with respect to cancer. In *Bathsheba's Breast*, a fascinating history

Table 6.3. Complementary Therapies That May Be Helpful	
Type of Therapy	*Ways in Which It May Be Helpful*
Mind-body therapies	Decrease anxiety and stress
	Improve sleep quality
	Improve quality of life
Acupuncture	Reduces nausea/vomiting from chemotherapy
	Decreases pain, especially musculoskeletal, headaches, and osteoarthritis
	Improves dry mouth (xerostomia) from radiation treatment
	Reduces hot flushes (also called hot flashes)*
	Reduces swelling from lymphedema*
	Improves sleep quality*
	Decreases anxiety and stress*
Massage	Decreases anxiety and stress
	Reduces pain, especially pain from muscle spasm

Source: G. Deng and B. Cassileth, "Complementary or Alternative Medicine in Cancer Care—Myths and Realities," *Nature Reviews Clinical Oncology* 10, no. 11 (November 2013): 656–64.

   Note: Just because these therapies may be helpful does not mean that they are safe for everyone to try. Talk to your doctor about what is right for you.

   *The scientific evidence is more controversial in these areas, but there are some studies that support these claims.

of breast cancer, James Olson writes about how frightened and vulnerable cancer patients have been exploited:

Desperation drives [cancer patients] into the hands of anyone with a promise and a smile. America is awash in cancer cons. . . . The quack treatment of choice in the 1950s was Harry Hoxey's Herbal Tonic. Hoxey set up shop in Dallas, Texas, in 1936, operating a "Cancer Clinic" to treat patients with an herbal tonic discovered decades before by his father on the family's Illinois farm. . . . [His father] marketed the cancer cure locally until 1919, when he died of cancer. His wife succumbed to the same disease two years later. Harry Hoxey inherited the "Herbal Tonic" and went into business operating the Hoxey Institute in Taylorville, Illinois. He soon expanded the product line, offering patients "black medicine." . . . As soon as the American Medical Association and state health officials caught up with him, Hoxey fled the state and started anew. He worked the con in Michigan, Iowa, and New Jersey before settling in Dallas. To get a sheepskin on the wall, he purchased an honorary doctorate of naturopathy. . . . With cruel skill, he played on the fears of his victims. . . . On a foundation of rhetorical overkill, he built a multimillion-dollar business, enjoying the political support of people like Senators Elmer Thomas of Oklahoma and William Langer of North Dakota. A number of right-wing political groups, such as the American Rally and the Christian Medical Research League, came to Hoxey's defense in 1950 when the Food and Drug Administration (FDA) went after him. After four years of litigation, the Supreme Court upheld the FDA's ban on Hoxey's Herbal Tonic, but by that time he had tricked tens of thousands of cancer patients into buying his worthless brew.

You may be thinking that this story is from the distant past and that such things could not happen nowadays. Not true. Duping cancer survivors happens all the time, and there is much needless suffering because of it. The FDA cautions consumers with this advice:

- If it sounds too good to be true, it probably is.
- Don't believe you have nothing to lose.
- Scientific (conventional) medicine is accountable.

If you aren't sure whether a person or treatment is legitimate, consider the following tips on how to identify quackery. Beware of

- any treatment or person claiming to heal a huge list of medical problems (for example, everything from ingrown toenails to cancer),
- promises of a "cure" for conditions without known cures (for example, arthritis),
- claims of "harmless" or "painless" procedures, and
- attacks on legitimate healthcare providers.

Beware of the unknown, such as

- the use of a "secret" formula, or
- any treatment for which there is no proven therapeutic effect (for example, a treatment that is discussed only in mass media and not in scientific literature).

Beware of demands for excessive commitments, such as:

- You need to follow a special diet or have treatment often and ongoing (this con often blames the failure of the treatment on the patient's inability to follow the rigorous plan).

COMPLEMENTARY THERAPIES AND HEALING

For a number of reasons complementary therapies may be beneficial in helping you to recover from cancer treatment. They may help reduce stress, improve sleep, relieve pain, and diminish symptoms of anxiety or depression. Some complementary therapies can help with treatment-related side effects, such as nausea or hot flashes. In some instances, they may also improve immune function. For example, studies have shown benefit from hypnosis for cancer pain and nausea; from relaxation therapy, music therapy, and massage for anxiety; and from acupuncture for nausea and pain.

Cancer patients most commonly try special dietary regimens, herbs, homeopathy, hypnosis, imagery, meditation, megadoses of vitamins, relaxation, and spiritual healing. Progressive muscle relaxation, imagery, hypnosis, prayer, and meditation are all reasonable to try. They may help reduce stress and pain and have essentially no side effects. Some treatments, such as massage and acupuncture, are usually fine to try, though in rare instances your doctor may not want you to use them. For instance, if your immune system has been suppressed by cancer treatment or if you are taking anticoagulants, then both massage and acupuncture may be unwise (check with your doctor). If you have extremely brittle bones from osteoporosis, then deep-tissue massage might not be the best treatment for you to try. Some doctors also recommend that you not have massage over an area where you had or have a tumor. Yoga is usually well tolerated unless extreme positions are used. Check with your doctor before beginning any exercise program.

Joseph Audette, MD, and I coauthored a chapter containing information about the healing effects of acupuncture in a book titled *Rehabilitation of Sports Injuries*. Here is an excerpt:

> The use of acupuncture by athletes to treat acute injuries is very common in Asia and Eastern Europe and is increasingly becoming an option in many Western nations. At the Winter Olympics in Japan in 1998, international exposure came when the acupuncturist in Nagano offered free treatments to Olympic athletes and officials, emphasizing that it is a drug-free way to treat injuries. Even more stunning was the near miraculous recovery in response to acupuncture by the Austrian, Hermann Maier. Maier won gold medals in the giant slalom and super G, 3 days following a dramatic fall and injury that occurred during the downhill competition. Maier mentioned to the press that the use of acupuncture to treat his shoulder and knee injuries following the fall helped him to recover so quickly.

As I indicated earlier, acupuncture is a legitimate integrative therapy that has scientific support for its use with some medical conditions and symptoms. Acupuncture may be used to treat some musculoskeletal conditions because of its pain-relieving (analgesic) effects and its effects on the immune system. The use of acupuncture in cancer patients may help with chemotherapy-related side effects such as nausea, vomiting, and pain. Acupuncture can also be tried in the posttreatment phase for residual surgical pain or other pain as well as to help heal musculoskeletal injuries. For example, one of my patients is a woman who had a mastectomy and developed significant *lymphedema*, a condition involving arm swelling that may occur after surgical exploration of the underarm lymph nodes. Because my patient was trying to protect the arm that had lymphedema, she overused her other arm and developed a common musculoskeletal overuse injury called *lateral epicondylitis* (also known as "tennis elbow"). Acupuncture may be helpful for lateral epicondylitis and is a reasonable remedy to prescribe.

Medical doctors are most concerned about patients who ingest herbal products or megadoses of vitamins or other supplements that are not regulated as drugs and therefore have not undergone rigorous scientific testing. These products can be purchased at drugstores and health food stores. In some instances, they might harm someone recovering from cancer treatment. Moreover, what these products actually contain and the quality of the preparation is variable. Extreme dietary regimens can also be hazardous to one's health and may inhibit healing.

Another problem with CAM treatments is that the people who are offering advice may have little or no training. For example, some states do not require any training or licensure to perform acupuncture. In one study, titled "Health Food Store Recommendations: Implications for Breast Cancer Patients," the authors investigated the advice given to women with breast cancer who visited thirty-four health food stores in a major Canadian city. Employees at the stores that were studied gave out quite a bit of advice—most of which was misleading and some of which was wrong and potentially very harmful. For example, the vast majority of consumers were not asked whether they were on any prescription medications, yet the employees felt confident recommending products to be ingested. There was no consistency in which products were suggested, and none of them had proven therapeutic value. Two employees suggested a possible cure with one of their products, and another employee told one woman to stop taking tamoxifen (a mainstream and proven treatment to help prevent breast cancer recurrence). These employees also offered advice on other "experts" to consult and suggested books for further reading. The authors noted, "This study also highlights the vulnerability of patients with breast cancer to potentially misleading information from health food employees. Advice presented by health food store employees was authoritative and could be misconstrued by patients as evidence-based, particularly when books are consulted or literature is provided on the products."

Of course, it is not just advice from health food store employees that one should be wary of. Well-meaning friends, neighbors, coworkers, and others often give advice about CAM treatments because they truly want to reach out to someone who is ill. As these therapies are further studied, much more information will be generated about which treatments will help people who have been diagnosed with cancer. An integrated healthcare approach is ideal, especially if we are able to use the best of all medical practices. Medical doctor Paul Brenner has an appreciation for many medical systems, and although he is an advocate of "holistic" medicine, he writes in *Buddha in the Waiting Room*, "Despite holism's many and correct emphases on responsibility, I have learned never to get sick at a holistic medical convention. Healers of every sort, shape, and size will pour out of the woodwork to save you from karmic death, nervous 'breakthroughs,' or lower back pain. They'll apply shiatsu, acupressure, acupuncture, rolfing, and polarity. And if none of these work, there's always a coffee-granule enema." Dr. Brenner goes on to say that the "cures" in New Age medicine are often suspect.

The field of integrative oncology is fascinating and offers some real possibilities for healing, but there is much research yet to be done. In the meantime, consider the recommendations listed in Tables 6.1 and 6.2, and if you want more information, refer to the resources listed in the "Resources for Complementary Therapies and Nutrition" section of the appendix. Although I suggest that all cancer survivors should remain firmly grounded in conventional medicine, even while exploring complementary therapies, I also appreciate many people's preference for a "holistic" approach. Using integrative therapies to help alleviate some symptoms such as pain, fatigue, stress, and so on may provide you with the greatest opportunity to heal well. One good resource for more information is the American Cancer Society's *Complete Guide to Complementary and Alternative Cancer Therapies.* This book can be found in many hospital cancer resource centers. Most of all, though, talk to your doctors about which therapies are safe and reasonable for you to try.

References

G. Deng G and B. Cassileth, "Integrative Oncology: An Overview," *American Society of Clinical Oncology Educational Book* (2014): 233–42.

"NIH Consensus Statement," *Acupuncture,* November 3–5, 1997, p. 19.

M. S. Goldstein, "Complementary and Alternative Medicine: Its Emerging Role in Oncology," *Journal of Psychosocial Oncology* 21 (2003): 4.

D. M. Eisenberg et al., "Unconventional Medicine in the United States—Prevalence, Costs, and Patterns of Use," *New England Journal of Medicine* 328 (1993): 246–52.

D. M. Eisenberg et al., "Trends in Alternative Medicine Use in the United States, 1990–1997: Results of a Follow-Up National Survey," *Journal of the American Medical Association* 280 (1998): 1570.

National Center for Complementary and Alternative Medicine, "What Is Complementary and Alternative Medicine (CAM)?," www.nccam.nih .gov/health/whatiscam, p. 3.

P. D. Hansten and J. R. Horn, *The Top 100 Drug Interactions: A Guide to Patient Management,* 5th ed. (Edmonds, WA: H and H, 2004).

J. Horn, personal communication, January 2005.

R. B. Saper et al., "Heavy Metal Content of Ayurvedic Herbal Medicine Products," *Journal of the American Medical Association* 292 (2004): 2868.

C. Horner, *Waking the Warrior Goddess: Dr. Christine Horner's Program to Protect against and Fight Breast Cancer* (North Bergen, NJ: Basic Health, 2005), pp. 26–27.

New York State Attorney General's Office, "A.G. Schneiderman Asks Major Retailers To Halt Sales Of Certain Herbal Supplements As DNA Tests Fail To Detect Plant Materials Listed On Majority Of Products Tested," press release, February 3, 2015, http://www.ag.ny.gov/press-re lease/ag-schneiderman-asks-major-retailers-halt-sales-certain-herbal -supplements-dna-tests

E. L. Davis, B. Oh, P. N. Butow, B. A. Mullan, and S. Clarke, "Cancer Patient Disclosure and Patient-Doctor Communication of Complementary and Alternative Medicine Use: A Systematic Review," *Oncologist* 17, no. 11 (2012): 1475–81.

C. W. Given et al., eds., *Evidence-Based Cancer Care and Prevention* (New York: Springer, 2003), p. 297.

W. A. Weiger et al., "Advising Patients Who Seek Complementary and Alternative Medical Therapies for Cancer," *Annals of Internal Medicine* 137 (2002): 893, 894.

J. S. Olson, *Bathsheba's Breast: Women, Cancer, and History* (Baltimore: Johns Hopkins University Press, 2002), pp. 83, 146–47.

J. K. Silver and J. Audette, "Pharmacological Agents and Acupuncture in Rehabilitation," in *Rehabilitation of Sports Injuries: Scientific Basis*, ed. Walter R. Frontera (Malden, MA: Blackwell Science, 2003), p. 198.

E. Mills, E. Ernst, R. Singh, C. Roos, and K. Wilson, "Health Food Store Recommendations: Implications for Breast Cancer Patients," *Breast Cancer Research* 5 (2003): R172.

P. Brenner, *Buddha in the Waiting Room* (Tulsa, OK: Council Oak Books, 2002), p. 110.

American Cancer Society, *Complete Guide to Complementary and Alternative Therapies*, Atlanta, GA: ACS, 2009.

{ CHAPTER 7 }

DANCE, SKIP,
AND WALK

Exercise Your Way Back to Health

I n 1929 an article in the journal *Medicine* offered this advice about how to help patients who had recently suffered a heart attack: "The nurse should be carefully instructed to do everything in her power to aid the patient in any physical activity so that all possible movements such as feeding himself or lifting himself in bed are spared. . . . Finally, the patient should be urged to spend at least six weeks, and preferably eight weeks or more, absolutely in bed."

Pioneering research beginning in the 1950s demonstrated that this was precisely the *wrong* way to treat someone who has suffered a heart attack. More than a half century later, it is now widely known that exercise has an important role in reducing the risk of having a heart attack and in helping people recover after having one.

You may wonder why I write about heart disease when this is a book about cancer. The reason is simple: research on the benefits of exercise in cancer is decades behind the research on the benefits exercise in heart disease. Ironically, at the same time doctors were recommending complete bed rest for heart patients during the 1920s, there were two studies done that suggested "hard muscular work" was important for cancer prevention. This theory wasn't further explored until the 1980s, when researchers again became interested in the effect of exercise on cancer prevention. In the interim, the studies that did focus on exercise and cancer examined the psychological perspective—no research was reported that looked at the effect of exercise on physiological or biological processes, and no studies assessed the impact of exercise on cancer recurrence.

The general idea of exercise as a panacea for health problems has ancient roots: around 400 BC Hippocrates advocated walking, slowly in the summer and quickly during winter months. During the nineteenth century, exercise was thought to build character and be good for the spirit. Some touted it as a moral obligation, and the term *muscular Christianity* came into use. In the early twentieth century, fitness became a fad. Sports historians refer to the 1920s as the "golden age of sport." A change occurred with the Depression, when people could no longer afford frivolities, including money spent on making their bodies look and feel good.

It was not until after World War II that exercise again took a prominent place in the lives of Americans. As *New York Times* reporter Gina Kolata points out in her book *Ultimate Fitness*, one leader of the next fitness movement (which continues unabated today) was Hans Kraus, a doctor specializing in physical medicine and rehabilitation, and his colleague Ruth Hirschland, who tested more than four thousand children and found that more than half of them were so unfit that they "failed to meet even a minimum standard required for health." They also tested European children and found less than 10 percent of them to be unfit. These reports drew national attention and started a new fitness craze. Soon scientists began to study intensely the health benefits of exercise, and savvy businesspeople tapped into a now multibillion-dollar industry.

More recently, exercise has been shown to help prevent some initial cancers from developing and also, in some cases, it may make a recurrence less likely once someone has already been diagnosed and treated. A review published by the American College of Sports Medicine evaluated eighty-five exercise studies in cancer survivors and found that, in general, exercise is safe during and after cancer treatment. Of course, check with your doctor about how best to exercise; safety is very important. This review also showed that moderate levels of exercise led to improvements in quality of life, anxiety, depression, fatigue, fitness, and strength. When it comes to whether exercise can help to avoid having cancer return and thereby improve survival rates, there are studies currently being conducted to try to answer this question; however, to date there are a number of small studies that suggest in some populations, such as people who have early-stage breast and colorectal cancer, exercise may positively impact survival.

While research on exercise and how it impacts cancer recovery and survival is still evolving, as I mentioned, there is more information about the psychological effects of exercise on people with cancer. Studies exploring this link have demonstrated that exercise definitely has a positive influence on mood and quality of life. Another important psychological finding is that, among people who have undergone physical changes with cancer treatment, those who are physically active report a greater sense of acceptance of their altered bodies.

Today, although there is still much research to be done on exercise in oncology populations, experts in oncology almost universally recognize that it is beneficial for people diagnosed with cancer before, during, and after treatment. As researchers continue their work, here are some of the questions they are currently studying:

Will exercise help prevent cancer?
Will exercise help prevent cancer recurrence?
Will exercise reduce side effects from cancer treatment?

Numerous early studies have been published, and many more are now trying to answer these questions and others.

Perhaps because breast cancer has been the most extensively studied type of cancer or possibly because of the disease itself, preliminary data are very positive with respect to physical activity in women with this diagnosis for all three of the issues: Exercise does seem to help prevent breast cancer from occurring in the first place. Exercise activity also appears to reduce the rate of its recurrence. For women who have had breast cancer, exercise has also been shown to decrease fatigue, the most prevalent and debilitating symptom cited during treatment. Dr. Carolyn Kaelin, a surgical oncologist, described the advice she gives to women diagnosed with breast cancer. In her book, *Living through Breast Cancer*, she has this to say about exercise:

> At their one-year checkup, the most common question my patients ask is, "What can I do for *myself* now?" All have had surgery. Some have had radiation or chemotherapy or both. Usually, their passage from the hands of one caring health professional to the next is finished, leaving an appeal in its wake. "Everyone has done something to me and for me. Now I want to do something for myself."
>
> At one time, I had few well-substantiated suggestions to offer. Now I have an excellent one. A growing number of research trials show that exercise is one factor within your control that, if you have been diagnosed with breast cancer, can make a very real difference to your life. What can it do? Exercise has been shown to help improve long-term survival, decrease the chance of breast cancer relapse, and minimize treatment-induced fatigue, bone loss, and muscle wasting. What's more, it can help you regain flexibility, strength, and endurance; ease certain side effects of treatment; and boost your quality of life.

How and why and to what extent exercise influences tumor growth is not well understood, but increasingly scientists are homing in on metabolic and inflammatory pathways that they believe are linked to cancer risk and prognosis. For example, obesity has been shown to be associated with resistance to our body's own insulin; we need insulin to keep blood sugar at a normal level. Similarly, obesity has been linked to low-grade chronic inflammation—this is something that isn't really noticeable but rather is tested in scientific studies. Exercise might improve both insulin resistance and inflammation, which can in turn make one's immune system stronger and better able to avoid or fight cancer. Exercise might reduce the availability of free radicals (components that may promote tumor growth) in the blood. Perhaps the amount of insulin, potentially a tumor growth factor, is reduced with exercise. There may be a direct effect on the tumor when blood is redistributed away from it to flow to skeletal muscle during exercise. Exercise may also affect hormones; some kinds of cancers, such as breast, endometrial, and testicular cancers, respond to hormones. There are many theories, and it is plausible that more than one will be found to be correct. We might also find that the reason exercise is helpful varies depending on the type of cancer. Eventually, all of these uncertainties will be sorted out.

Obviously there is much we don't know about exercise and cancer, but one thing we do know is that exercise assists in getting people ready for cancer treatment, helping them to tolerate chemotherapy and other therapies and fast-tracking their ability to heal. There are a few exceptions, but unless you have a serious heart or lung problem, exercise will likely offer you real advantages as you begin, undergo, or recover from cancer treatment. Some of the benefits of exercise include improving strength and endurance, reducing fatigue and facilitating good sleep, decreasing muscle soreness and other body pains, and, of course, improving mood and optimism (see Table 7.1). Exercise is one of the least risky and most beneficial treatment options doctors have to offer cancer survivors. It is true that in exceedingly rare instances, a person may suffer a fatal heart attack or stroke while exercising, but in general people can safely exercise after getting clearance from their doctors. You may be concerned about the risk of injuries; keep in mind that individuals who are sedentary have a higher risk not only of heart disease and stroke if they *don't* exercise, but also of conditions such as chronic low-back pain. In short, as you become more physically fit, you will in all likelihood have less pain and improved health.

Table 7.1. General Benefits of Exercise	
Improves heart and lung function	Enhances immune system function
Reduces the risk of serious heart problems	Promotes a positive outlook
Increases metabolic rate	Reduces stress, anxiety, and depression
Enhances strength	Lessens fatigue
Lowers cholesterol levels	Contributes to better sleep
Strengthens bones	Improves quality of life
Helps to control blood sugar levels	
Improves lean body mass and helps to control weight	

Energetics: The Combined Effect of Diet and Exercise

One of the most important new areas of research is looking at the relationship between diet and exercise versus just evaluating diet or exercise alone. As I mentioned previously, the term for this is *energetics*. Expanding on my earlier example, a woman is diagnosed with breast cancer and is a little overweight and sedentary with a poor diet. She may benefit the most from diet and exercise working synergistically. Consider these three scenarios:

1. She doesn't exercise or change her diet and her weight stays the same.
2. She begins to exercise but doesn't change her diet. Her weight stays the same, but she develops more lean body mass (muscle).
3. She begins to exercise and significantly improves her diet, too. Her weight stays the same.

Obviously, the best option for her health is the third one. We know this because we have information about her weight, diet, and exercise. If we knew only about her weight, we might be led to believe that her health didn't change. And it's fairly easy to surmise that if she makes two positive changes—exercise and diet—it's better than either one of them alone.

As I've mentioned, prehabilitation can help get cancer survivors physically and emotionally ready for upcoming surgery and other treatments. In a review of prehabilitation studies that I wrote with my colleague Dr. Jennifer Baima, we discussed the concept of "multimodal" prehabilitation—which essentially means that there is more than one intervention. Multimodal prehabilitation is an important topic because researchers believe that it works better than exercise alone. For example, Dr. Franco Carli has published multiple prehabilitation studies in colorectal cancer survivors. In one of the studies, he and his team looked at a trimodal approach. This approach consisted of nutritional protein supplementation, using specific stress reduction strategies and exercise. I've talked to Dr. Carli about his work, and he firmly believes that these three interventions work much better together than any one of them would work alone. Furthermore, in one of his recent studies, he compared two groups of colorectal patients and found that the group that had both prehabilitation and postoperative rehabilitation did better physically than the group that just had the postoperative rehabilitation. This study was exciting, because it suggests that the earlier you get started, the better.

The studies on both prehabilitation and energetics are evolving, and over time we will have more information about how they can impact health outcomes in cancer survivors. For example, there are fifteen new studies being conducted as part of something called the Transdisciplinary Research on Energetics and Cancer initiative. The results of these studies will be fascinating and almost certainly will demonstrate that the combined effects of improving your diet and physical activity level will be better than focusing on just one of them.

BASIC COMPONENTS OF AN EXERCISE REGIMEN

For the best results, include all three main exercise components in your routine. An exercise program should

1. improve strength,
2. improve flexibility, and
3. improve cardiovascular fitness.

A helpful mnemonic for a good exercise regimen is FITT, which stands for

Frequency
Intensity
Time
Type

FITT will be involved in any well-written physical therapy prescription. So, let's say that you have just completed chemotherapy and want to begin to rebuild your cardiovascular endurance. If you don't have any serious heart or lung problems, then a reasonable exercise prescription would state how often you should exercise, what intensity level you should maintain, how much time you should spend on an activity, and what specific types of exercise you are to do.

Typically when a doctor writes a formal physical therapy prescription, the patient takes it to a physical therapist. Many people begin or resume exercising without physical therapy, too, though it can be a great way to get started. What I recommend is that you first talk to your primary care physician or your oncologist about how and when to begin exercising. Your doctor may recommend that you begin on your own, that you go to a physical therapist or fitness professional for guidance, or that you consult with a physiatrist (a doctor who specializes in rehabilitation) for help in managing your cancer recovery process. No matter how you begin, you can use the FITT principle to guide you.

Most doctors do not have much formal training in how to prescribe exercise as a method to help people heal. (Major exceptions are physiatrists and orthopedists.) The reason they don't is that there is so much to know in medicine; it is impossible to be an expert in every aspect of health care. But whether or not your oncologist and your primary care physician know a lot about exercise, they are usually excellent resources and can either help you begin to exercise or can refer you to an oncology rehabilitation specialist who will guide you.

Also please look at Table 7.2, which is a list of therapeutic measures that can be helpful or potentially harmful to people with cancer. The American Physical Therapy Association publishes guidelines on the use of modalities in oncology rehabilitation. Its guidelines are not necessarily based on research, though, but rather on assumptions and precautions that health professionals believe are reasonable. There isn't much research done to test the harmfulness of various measures because it would never be reasonable to design a study in which the anticipated consequences would be harmful to the participants. Therefore, the modalities that might not be safe for people with cancer listed in Table 7.2 are some that survivors should generally avoid because they *might* be harmful.

EXERCISE TESTING

The American Heart Association and the American College of Sports Medicine have both issued formal exercise guidelines that include ad-

Table 7.2. Safe and Unsafe Physical Modalities

Modalities That Might Not Be Safe for People with Cancer

Superficial heat (for example, hot packs) and deep heat (for example, ultrasound): Usually not used directly over a tumor site because of the theoretical concern that increased blood flow may encourage tumor growth. However, this issue is controversial.

Massage / manipulation / percussion / soft tissue mobilization: Generally avoided in the area of a malignancy. This is another controversial issue; there is also the suggestion that massage may be helpful in various ways, including enhancing immune function. For further information see chapter 10.

Neuromuscular stimulation, transcutaneous electrical nerve stimulation (TENS), and interferential stimulation: Generally avoided in the area of a malignancy.

Mechanical traction of the spine: Usually avoided in people who have had cancer in or near their spine.

Modalities Considered Safe for People with Cancer

Cryotherapy (for example, cold packs)
Iontophoresis
Biofeedback

vice on when tests (such as a cardiac stress test) should be administered before beginning an exercise program. These guidelines are generally focused on individuals over 40 years of age, and although they are useful, they are not meant for people who are undergoing or have recently finished treatment for cancer. The guidelines do not take into account the reasons cardiovascular exercise might need to be limited for these individuals. For example, a person with cancer might be anemic, so that the body has a reduced ability to deliver oxygen to the muscles. Or the person might have developed one of the unusual heart side effects from a chemotherapy drug such as Adriamycin. It is because of such possibilities that I advise *all* cancer survivors to talk with their doctors prior to starting an exercise program and learn how they can safely proceed. If for some reason there is a delay in getting an appointment and you don't have any known heart or lung problems, then you can usually safely begin a gentle walking and stretching program.

A doctor who is guiding a patient in beginning an exercise regimen may ask the person to have some formal tests, such as an electrocardiogram (EKG) or a cardiac stress test (usually done on a treadmill or with an upper-extremity bike, for safety in people who aren't steady on a treadmill). The physician may suggest physical or occupational therapy, particularly for a person who is very unfit physically or has other medical issues such as postoperative musculoskeletal pain, delayed wound healing or uncomfortable scarring, or underlying health problems such as diabetes or heart disease. The therapist might be asked to monitor vital signs during exercise: blood pressure, heart rate, and respiratory rate. At my center, we also monitor the blood oxygen levels during exercise, by using a pulse oximeter that clips onto the person's finger.

BEFORE GETTING STARTED

Before starting an exercise regimen, be sure to talk to your doctor about whether you can exercise, and also get information about what types of exercises you can do, how hard you should push yourself, what you should avoid, and what problems you may encounter. If you have had surgery, your doctor will probably not want you to exercise within a month or so of the operation. Of course the type of surgery makes a difference. If you have had a melanoma removed from your skin, that incision will typically heal more quickly than, say, an abdominal or a chest surgery. Most doctors encourage their patients to exercise while in chemotherapy or radiation treatment unless they are at risk for certain complications—internal bleeding due to low red blood cell levels or infection due to low white blood cell levels, for example.

As part of your mental preparation, decide that you will exercise regularly. Using physical activity as a healing tool involves the key component of making exercise a habit—something you do without giving it much thought. Starting any new habit takes concentration and planning, but before long it becomes simple and routine. You may enjoy exercising more if you join a class such as yoga or jazz dance. Hospitals and other organizations such as the YMCA often offer these types of classes for people with health concerns, so you may want to contact your local facilities. Meeting a friend to go for a walk might help you overcome inertia. Do not feel guilty if you take a day, a week, or a month off. Guilt leads to stress, and stress isn't good for your body or spirit. So, if you stop exercising for a while, rather than let guilt or worry weigh you down, simply plan a time when you can get back on track and then congratulate yourself for doing so.

Some people consult fitness professionals such as a personal trainer as they start or maintain an exercise program. One benefit of fitness professionals is that they provide excellent help to keep you motivated to exercise. Good fitness professionals, especially exercise physiologists, are also very skilled in teaching the correct way to perform specific exercises. Be aware, however, that fitness professionals have expertise in exercise but are not the same as rehabilitation professionals such as physical therapists who can treat physical impairments. Some of them may offer advice about how to treat injuries and illnesses, but in doing so they go beyond the scope of their training. Again, I advise people with cancer to ask their doctors and other rehabilitation professionals, such as physical therapists, about their health concerns.

GETTING STARTED

Here are some specific tips that may be helpful as you set off on your own exercise program.

As you exercise, it can be fun and motivating to track your progress. If you wrote down exercise goals after reading chapter 2, refer to them now. (If you didn't record any goals then, consider jotting some down now.) Start an exercise log and record the date, the activity you do, and how you feel when you finish. List your exercise goals in the log, and show how you will track them. From time to time, look back at earlier entries in your log to see how far you've come. You can also apply the FITT principle, which means that you record in your log frequency (how often you exercise), intensity (how hard you exercise), time (how long you exercise), and type (what kind of exercise you do).

Established guidelines suggest that adults aged 18–64 years should engage in at least 150 minutes, or two and a half hours, per week of moderate-intensity exercise, or 75 minutes of vigorous exercise. Adults over the age of 65 years should also follow these recommendations if possible, but they may be limited by chronic health conditions such as arthritis. When you are exercising with moderate intensity, you can usually talk but not sing. It's a good idea to calculate the range for your target heart rate (THR) and try to keep your heart rate within that range when you exercise. When you begin, you may want to stay close to the lower number in the range; as you get stronger and have more endurance, you can push yourself a bit harder and work at the upper end of your range. Record your range in your log, so you can easily refer to it. See Table 7.3 for a simple calculation to find your THR. You can monitor your heart rate by taking your pulse at the wrist or the neck. Another way that is inexpensive and fun is to use a heart-rate monitor. You can get a monitor at your local sporting goods store and from many online retailers.

Table 7.3. Monitoring Your Target Heart Rate (THR)

A heart-rate monitor, available at your local sporting goods store, can be a fun way to help you get a good cardiac workout. Some general guidelines are as follows: Most people's resting heart rate is usually between 60 and 90 beats per minute. For young adults, the maximum recommended heart rates with exercise are around 190–200, and for middle-aged and older adults they are generally 140–160. Your THR is the rate you should aim for when you are doing cardiovascular exercise. If you have done some exercise testing, you may have been told what your THR is, or you may have been given a target range. If you don't know your THR, you can figure it by using this formula:

Maximum heart rate (MHR) = 220 − your age
Target heart rate (lower limit) = 0.6 × MHR
Target heart rate (upper limit) = 0.8 × MHR

So, if you are 50 years old, your MHR is 170 (220 − 50 = 170). This means that the lower limit of your THR is 0.6 × 170 = 102 and the upper limit is 0.8 × 170 = 136. You can round these numbers off and use 100–135 as your THR range, which means that you try to exercise at least hard enough to raise your heart rate above 100, but you don't let it exceed 135. THR goals can be a bit higher in people who are very fit and a bit lower in people who have heart conditions or take blood pressure medications.

{ Before and After Cancer Treatment }

Weigh yourself and calculate your body mass index (BMI). This is a great measurement to track. The easiest way to do it is to go to a website such as the one for the Centers for Disease Control and Prevention (www.cdc.gov/nccdphp/dnpa/bmi/calc-bmi.htm) and just plug in your height and weight. Or you can do the math yourself (check Table 7.4 for the formula). Record the results in your log and check it once a month. Here are the guidelines to help you decide whether you need to gain or lose weight:

BMI	Weight Status
Below 18.5	Underweight
18.5–24.9	Normal
25.0–29.9	Overweight
30.0 and Above	Obese

Perform a 6-minute walk (or run) test and measure how far you can go. You can do the test on a track where you know the distance around the perimeter, or you can do it in your neighborhood and then find out how far you went by driving the same route and checking the car's mileage tracking device or use Google maps or another app. Record the distance in your log and repeat the test monthly to monitor your progress.

Buy a pedometer and count your steps. This simple and inexpensive device gives you another way to monitor your progress and keep yourself motivated (see Table 7.5). (You can raise your activity level with a pedometer even if you are not in a formal exercise program.)

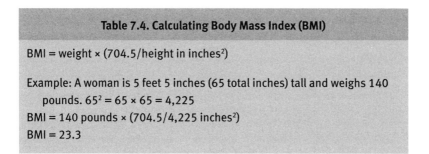

Table 7.4. Calculating Body Mass Index (BMI)

BMI = weight × (704.5/height in inches²)

Example: A woman is 5 feet 5 inches (65 total inches) tall and weighs 140 pounds. 65² = 65 × 65 = 4,225
BMI = 140 pounds × (704.5/4,225 inches²)
BMI = 23.3

Table 7.5. Track Your Steps

Use a pedometer to measure how your endurance is increasing. You can purchase one inexpensively at most sporting goods stores or at www .walk4life.com and use it to find out how many steps you take either during your aerobic exercise session or throughout the day. One mile is about 2,000 steps. Try it out and see how many steps you take from the time you wake up until the time you go to bed each day for three days. Record your results in a journal or a log. Attempt to increase your steps per day by 10 percent each week. If you are currently taking 2,000 steps, then your goal for next week would be 2,200, and your goal for next month would be 2,800. You may advance a little slower or faster; it's not something to worry about. The 10-percent-per-week rule is just a guideline. I usually recommend that people progress to 5,000–10,000 steps per day.

CARDIOVASCULAR EXERCISE

Mark Twain, a literary genius in many respects, had it all wrong when it came to exercise. In a speech he made for his seventieth birthday, he said, "I have never taken any exercise, except sleeping and resting, and I never intend to take any. Exercise is loathsome." If you have never exercised regularly or if you have decreased your activity level during or following treatment, you might think it will be difficult to fit exercise into your life. We can forgive Twain for denouncing exercise because he didn't have the perspective that a cancer survivor has nor did he have access to the knowledge we have today regarding the importance of exercise in general. Perhaps if he had known all that we know, he would have started exercising—even at 70 he could still have reaped the benefits.

Cardiovascular, or aerobic, exercise is any activity that you can sustain for several minutes or longer (see Table 7.6 for examples). In this form of exercise, you are primarily engaging type 1 muscle fibers, which are the "slow oxidative" or "slow twitch" fibers that function by utilizing oxygen. Aerobic exercises also make use of several muscle groups—not just one group—over and over again. For example, cycling, swimming, walking, and dancing involve more than one muscle group. Cardiovascular exercises are great for improving your level of endurance. If you regularly perform an exercise of this type, you will find that you can

Table 7.6. Cardiovascular Exercises	
Walking	Dancing
Hiking	Working out with an aerobics class
Jogging	Jumping rope
Rowing	Using stair-climbing, elliptical, or
Cycling	spinning machines
Roller-skating or ice-skating	Cross-country skiing
Roller-blading	Snowshoeing
Swimming	

keep doing it for longer and longer periods and usually at increased rates. Moreover, you will likely notice that you have less fatigue in your daily activities—not only when you are exercising.

Many recovering people can begin to exercise on their own by simply returning gradually to what they used to do. (Studies show that people who go through treatment for cancer often become very sedentary during their therapy and then don't return to their former activity levels.) During and just after my chemotherapy, my ability to perform aerobic exercise varied a lot. On "good days" I could easily walk 1–2 miles in my neighborhood. On "bad days" I would get to the final part of my walk, where there was a small incline, and ask my husband to help me finish (he would gently pull or push me). I would start out fine and then fatigue much more quickly and more profoundly than I had in the past. It was hard for me to predict what I could do because I didn't have the same end-of-exercise stamina. Still, I did the best I could and kept going for my walks.

Since I live in Massachusetts, where the weather often prohibits outdoor exercise, I would also exercise on my elliptical machine every time I talked on the phone. I have a handset with a speaker phone, so when the phone rang, I would answer it, start my elliptical trainer, and begin to exercise and talk simultaneously. This system worked well because my conversations were usually short (5–15 minutes) and talking kept me entertained. I would do this routine several times a day, and the minutes added up. As I got stronger and had more endurance, I could stay on the machine for 30–45 minutes and get a full workout.

The American Cancer Society recommends, for the aerobic component of an exercise program, that a person aim to work up to a moderate-intensity (or higher) regimen for 30 minutes five days a week. If you can comfortably tolerate 45-minute workouts, they might give you some added benefit over 30-minute sessions. It has been suggested, however, that in some cancers overexercising may be detrimental to immune function. This matter is not well understood. There are no formal recommendations about the *maximum* level of exercise that cancer survivors should achieve. What I tell my patients is that if they exercised regularly prior to cancer treatment, they should try to return to the same level of exercise. If they were relatively sedentary prior to treatment, then the goal is to exercise *regularly* rather than exercise for a long time in a given session.

If you are becoming overly fatigued from the cardiovascular component of your exercise program, consider trying one or more of the following suggestions:

- Employ the concept of interval training; that is, alternate periods of performing the activity with rest breaks. This way you establish a work-rest cycle that helps to provide you with the necessary energy to do the exercise. Keep in mind that the longer the rest phase, the greater your ability to recover between cycles.
- Decrease the intensity of the activity (for example, walk or cycle at a slower rate).
- Decrease the duration of your session (if you are exercising continuously for 30 minutes, try going for 20 minutes instead).
- Decrease the frequency of your sessions (if you are taking a walk daily, you can try switching to every other day to see whether giving yourself a break will help you to have more endurance on the days you do walk).

BUILDING STRENGTH

Strength training has health benefits for everyone, but it can be particularly helpful for a person recovering from cancer and its treatment (see Table 7.7). Strengthening exercises can do much more than just help you lift heavier items. For example, one day I was talking to my son,

Table 7.7. Benefits of Strength Training

Improved strength and overall fitness	Better balance and coordination
Increased lean body mass	Less effort to perform work and
Stronger bones	home activities
Better immune function	Improved sense of well-being
Improved metabolism	

who had just gone through a growth spurt, about the need to improve his posture. He looked at me and said, not unkindly, "Mom, *you* used to be all bent over." Touché. It was true. When I was undergoing cancer treatment, I was in pain and often unintentionally hunched over. My posture improved dramatically with strength training in my upper body.

Strengthening or resistance exercises involve short bursts of muscular activity; therefore, the muscle fibers that are called on tend to be type 2. Muscles contain both type 1 and type 2 fibers, though in different amounts from one muscle to another. When you perform strengthening exercises, you are not utilizing oxidative pathways, which rely on oxygen as a primary source of energy. Instead, these are anaerobic exercises. There are a couple of concepts in strength training that you may hear discussed. According to the "size principle," if you lift too light a load compared to what you are able to lift, then you will be working more type 1 fibers than type 2 fibers. You cannot improve your strength very much that way. The other concept, called the "overload principle," is that to build strength, you must overload the muscle. Understanding these two principles will help you to avoid perhaps the most common error in strength training—lifting a load that is too light and doing too many repetitions. Strength is built when you tax your muscles and do only a few repetitions. We call this a "high load, low rep" program. A good way to find out how much you can lift is to determine the largest amount of weight you can lift just one time (this is a one-repetition maximum, or 1 RM) and then how much weight you can lift ten consecutive times (this is a 10 RM). We use these values to advise people how much they should lift to begin a strength-training program. The following is an easy strength-training formula that begins with lighter weights and increases the amount of weight (or resistance) during the same session. This approach to strength training (one of several) is called *progressive resistance exercise* and is one way to do strength training.

Figure out how much weight you can lift 10 times. This will be your 10 RM. Then begin your session and advance as follows:

Set 1. Start the first set of ten repetitions with 50 percent of your 10 RM (if your 10 RM weight is 10 pounds, then begin with 5 pounds and lift it ten times. Generally it is better and safer to begin this process by using an exercise weight machine rather than free weights, although free weights are fine for lighter loads and for individuals who have been properly trained to use heavier free weights).

Set 2. Rest for 1–2 minutes (or longer if you need to), and then do the second set with 60 percent of your 10 RM (or 6 pounds if your 10 RM is 10).

Set 3. Again rest for 1–2 minutes and perform the final set with 80 percent of the 10 RM (8 pounds in our example).

You will want to work on strengthening your entire body, and this is usually done best by working on several muscle groups during one session. You may want to cross-train and alternate the muscles you work on—so that you are not working on everything all at once. Strength training is generally done less often than cardiovascular exercise (2–3 times a week rather than 5–7 times a week) because it is best to allow for a recovery period.

IMPROVING FLEXIBILITY

Flexibility exercises often have a Cinderella complex. They tend to be the neglected part of an exercise regimen. Yet, when they are done regularly, they can enhance a person's well-being. Cardiovascular and strengthening exercises are the *most* important for healing, however, so if your time and energy are too limited to include all three types of exercise, you should concentrate on those two.

Ironically, sometimes even athletes who have had a lot of excellent coaching fail to stretch—and pay a price for it. For example, a nationally ranked long jumper came to see me about her back pain. She had been suffering for weeks and had quit working out with her team. During the visit she asked me whether she should take the year off and "red shirt" to save a year of eligibility. After reviewing her previous workup, including a magnetic resonance imaging study (MRI) of her low back, which did not reveal any reason for her pain, I performed a physical examination. When I noticed that she had very tight hamstring muscles (a problem that often contributes to low-back pain), I asked her about the flexibility part of her exercise regimen. She replied, "Oh, I hardly ever stretch." I explained that while speed and strength are tremendous assets in an athlete, flexibility is also vital to perform optimally and to avoid injury.

You can begin to stretch in a number of different ways. One way is to do a series of gentle stretching exercises at home. When you stretch, you should feel an uncomfortable, but not painful, sensation. Often people describe this as a "burning" feeling. If you don't feel anything, chances are that you are not obtaining a good stretch. If you feel pain, then you are overstretching and risking injury to the muscle or tendon. Stretching works best if you do it gently, without rocking or bobbing up and down, and hold it for at least 10–15 seconds. Stretching exercises are often done after a cardiovascular workout when your body is warmed up. Some people do them before aerobic exercise because the stretching enhances their agility and balance. If you do several stretches after every cardiovascular workout, then you are on the right track.

Yoga and Tai Chi are great ways to stretch, especially for beginners. I don't recommend some of the more advanced yoga positions because they put a tremendous strain on the muscles, tendons, and ligaments. Patients often ask me whether they have to do all of the stretches in a yoga or Tai Chi class. The answer is no. You should do only what feels comfortable to you and doesn't cause you pain. I find that people tend to be smart and intuitive about their bodies. Yoga and other instructors can be helpful, too. Talk to them about what is bothering you, as they often have excellent suggestions to avoid discomfort. However, if it doesn't feel right to you, don't do it.

Going through cancer treatment often leads to musculoskeletal or other problems that can limit one's ability to exercise. Surgery can cause residual pain for weeks or even months. Scar tissue can reduce the range of motion of joints. Chemotherapy and radiation can also cause side effects that place limitations on exercise. For example, Carol is a 50-year-old woman who came to see me after she was diagnosed with breast cancer. Initially Carol underwent a right mastectomy combined with breast reconstruction. A few months later she had breast reduction surgery on her unaffected side to make her breasts the same size. Following this operation, the pathology reports revealed that Carol had cancer in her left breast as well, so she elected to have a left mastectomy with another reconstruction procedure, combined with chemotherapy and radiation.

When I initially saw Carol in consultation more than a year later, she was complaining of tightness and pressure across her chest, and she couldn't fully raise her arms overhead. She also had pain in both arms and in her neck. Her symptoms were due to a combination of scar tissue from the surgeries, contracted soft tissues around her chest and arms because she had not stretched during radiation treatment, and frozen shoulders because she had not lifted her arms overhead (it was too painful). I was surprised to learn that she had had more than 130 visits with a physical therapist over the previous year, with little improvement.

After examining Carol, I wrote specific orders for physical therapy at my center. I knew the physical therapist assigned to treat her was highly skilled and would be able to help her in a short time. Two months later, after thirteen physical therapy visits, Carol came for a follow-up appointment. She informed me that she was 80 percent better and happily lifted her arms overhead without any trouble. Her chest and arm pain was gone, and there was only a bit of residual chest tightness from the scar tissue. This case is an extreme one, but it is a true story that highlights the need for cancer survivors with specific issues to work with healthcare providers who are experts. See Table 7.8 for general suggestions on exercise adaptations for specific medical conditions and

Table 7.8. Exercise Adaptations for Medical Problems

Arthritis

To avoid stress on your joints, choose non-weight-bearing cardiovascular exercises, for example, cycling and swimming. Taking breaks will help to minimize pain. You can strengthen the muscles around painful joints by doing isometric exercises (exercises that do not involve movement). If you have arthritis in your knees, for example, lie on your back, raise your leg 1 foot off the ground, and hold it for 30 seconds, with or without an ankle weight. This exercise strengthens your quadriceps muscles but places minimal stress on the knee joints.

Diabetes

Cardiovascular exercises may lower a person's blood sugar level, so if you have diabetes, your blood sugar needs to be monitored carefully. A lower load and more repetitions are recommended for diabetics doing strengthening exercises.

Back Pain

Lumbar stabilization exercises are recommended to improve core (middle-of-the-body) muscle strength and flexibility. Generally avoid high-load strengthening exercises.

Osteoporosis

Weight-bearing exercises, including both aerobic and muscle-strengthening exercises, help to strengthen bones. Of note is that swimming and water aerobic exercises, while good for your heart, do not strengthen your bones because they are non-weight bearing.

Hypertension (High Blood Pressure)

Strengthening is best done using a lower load and more repetitions. A person with hypertension should avoid isometric exercises (which involve a sustained muscle contraction rather than moving the muscle through its range of motion, such as in a biceps curl).

Table 7.9 for help with cancer-related exercise issues. Table 7.10 contains advice on when to stop exercising and when to avoid it altogether.

Exercise is a crucial part of healing and is one of the most important factors in the process. However, not all exercise is created equal, and many cancer survivors have physical impairments that need to be addressed by rehabilitation professional prior to exercising on their own or with a fitness professional. Therefore, it's important to incorporate

Table 7.9. Problems Cancer Survivors May Encounter

Lymphedema

Lymphedema is the swelling of a limb (seen most frequently in people with breast cancer who have swelling of an arm after some of their underarm lymph nodes are removed during surgery). The swelling is caused by extra lymph fluid that collects in the limb as a result of disruption in the lymph nodes and the flow through them. In the past, it was believed that exercise, especially strenuous exercises done with the affected limb, might cause or promote this problem. But the research on lymphedema and exercise is inconclusive; it may be that exercise actually helps protect people from getting lymphedema. And, for those who have it, exercise may improve the symptoms. I have patients with lymphedema who race dragon boats using paddles, and this exercise doesn't seem to make their symptoms worse. Besides, they are more physically fit than if they were not exercising, and I believe the exercise helps them emotionally as well.

My advice if you have or are at risk for lymphedema is to ask your doctor to recommend the best types of exercise for you and what precautions you should take (maybe wearing an elasticized arm or leg sleeve while you exercise). I generally advise my patients to avoid strenuous weight lifting, although light weights (for example, 5 RM, or 50 percent of the maximum you can lift) should be all right.

Ostomy

Having an ostomy shouldn't prevent you from exercising. The main precaution for a person with an ostomy is to avoid contact sports because a blow could result in injury to the stoma and because the pouching system could slip or become dislodged. Weight lifting can result in a hernia at the stoma. Strengthening exercises can still be performed, but I would advise working with a physical therapist to develop a strengthening program that minimizes intra-abdominal pressure. Swimming is not a problem as long as the ostomy is sealed.

Surgery

Surgical wounds will lay down the first layers of healing cells within twenty-four hours, but most doctors don't recommend beginning exercise until the incision appears to be well sealed (even though it doesn't look completely healed), the stitches or staples are out, and at least a few weeks have passed since the surgery (often the exercise start date is 4–6 weeks after the date of the operation). If there is evidence of infection or if you are undergoing additional cancer treatments (for example, chemotherapy), there may be a delay in the healing of the incision and the beginning of an exercise regimen.

Infection Risk

During chemotherapy and some immunotherapy treatments, a person's blood counts may dip to a level that puts the person at risk for infection. In that case, it is wise to avoid public places (including gyms, spas, and so forth). Your doctor may advise you not to exercise at all until your cell counts come up to a safe level.

Skin Changes

Many cancer treatments make the skin more fragile. In this situation you can help to protect your skin by wearing comfortable clothing (generally 100 percent cotton is best) and by avoiding excessive sweating, which may further irritate your skin. It may also be helpful to wrap an irritated area with a gauze pad or bandage. In general, avoid chlorinated pools if you are undergoing radiation therapy and have injury to your skin.

Scarring

Scars from surgery may interfere with exercising effectively because of pain or because they restrict the range of motion of a joint. In such a case, usually supervised physical or occupational therapy is advisable.

Pain

Pain may be related to postoperative healing, surgical scarring, medications that may cause muscle aches, and so on. For some types of pain, it is safe to "push through" it. But in certain conditions it is better to avoid making the pain symptoms worse, because doing so will exacerbate the underlying problem. If you are experiencing pain, talk to your doctor about the cause and treatment and whether the pain will affect your ability to exercise. Again, supervised physical or occupational therapy may be beneficial in dealing with pain.

Deconditioning

Exercise is usually safe to do both during and after cancer treatment. It helps to avoid deconditioning (loss of physical fitness). However, in the midst of treatment and even after cancer therapy has finished, you may quickly lose muscle strength and begin to feel generally tired. If fatigue and lack of endurance are making it difficult for you to exercise, then try the suggestions listed in the chapter (interval training, sitting to exercise, and using a lower load for strength training).

(continued)

Table 7.9. (continued)

Dizziness and Feeling Unstable

If you are experiencing these symptoms, talk to your doctor. Dizziness and an unstable feeling may be caused by low blood counts, hormonal changes, general deconditioning, medication side effects, and more. If your doctor tells you it is safe to exercise despite these symptoms, then you can choose exercises that are done either seated or lying down to minimize your symptoms and reduce the risk of falling and injuring yourself.

Table 7.10. When Exercise Might Not Be Good for You

Stop exercising immediately and report these symptoms to your doctor if you experience

  Excessive fatigue or shortness of breath
  Heart palpitations
  Chest, jaw, or arm pain
  Dizziness or light-headedness

Avoid exercise if you

  Recently had surgery and haven't been cleared by your doctor
  Have any type of infection, including infection in a surgical incision or an upper respiratory infection
  Have uncontrolled pain, nausea, or other treatment side effects
  Feel dizzy or unstable and haven't been cleared by your doctor to exercise with these symptoms
  Have a fever greater than 100 degrees
  Had chemotherapy within the past 24 hours (check with your doctor on when to exercise following chemotherapy or other treatments)
  Have low blood cell counts (it is up to your doctor to determine safe levels—general guidelines are listed below)

Avoid exercise if cell counts are less than

Platelet count	50,000
Hemoglobin	10
White blood cell count	3,000
Absolute granulocyte count	2,500

exercise safely and appropriately with other healing interventions and to get expert advice about how to do this. The good news is that there is an increasing amount of information suggesting that exercise can help to prevent cancer in the first place and perhaps to prevent a relapse. Moreover, improvements in diet and exercise—energetics—may exponentially increase healing over either one of these alone. By exercising regularly, you are helping yourself to heal as well as possibly preventing new cancers from developing and decreasing the likelihood that cancer will come back. At the same time, you are lowering your risk of developing the most common life-threatening medical condition—heart disease. The benefits of exercise are enormous and the risks very small when it is done under a doctor's supervision.

References

S. A. Levine and C. L. Brown, "Coronary Thrombosis," *Medicine* 8 (1929): 1570.

G. Kolata, *Ultimate Fitness* (New York: Picador, 2003), pp. 41–42.

K. H. Schmitz, K. S. Courneya, C. Matthews, et al., "American College of Sports Medicine Roundtable on Exercise Guidelines for Cancer Survivors," *Medicine & Science in Sports & Exercise* 42 (2010): 1409–26.

C. Kaelin, *Living Through Breast Cancer* (New York: McGraw-Hill, 2005), p. 243.

J. K. Silver and J. Baima, "Cancer Prehabilitation: An Opportunity to Decrease Treatment-Related Morbidity, Increase Cancer Treatment Options, and Improve Physical and Psychological Health Outcomes," *American Journal of Physical Medicine & Rehabilitation* 92, no. 8 (August 2013): 715–27.

C. Gillis, C. Li, L. Lee, R. Awasthi, B. Augustin, A. Gamsa, A. S. Liberman, B. Stein, P. Charlebois, L. S. Feldman, and F. Carli, "Prehabilitation versus Rehabilitation: A Randomized Control Trial in Patients Undergoing Colorectal Resection for Cancer," *Anesthesiology* 121, no. 5 (November 2014): 937–47.

R. E. Patterson, G. A. Colditz, F. B. Hu, K. H, Schmitz, R. S. Ahima, R. C. Brownson, K. R. Carson, J. E. Chavarro, L. A. Chodosh, S. Gehlert, et al., "The 2011–2016 Transdisciplinary Research on Energetics and Cancer (TREC) Initiative: Rationale and Design," *Cancer Causes Control* 24, no. 4 (April 2013): 695–704.

C. L. Rock, C. Doyle, W. Demark-Wahnefried, J. Meyerhardt, K. S. Courneya, A. L. Schwartz, E. V. Bandera, K. K. Hamilton, B. Grant, M. McCullough, et al., "Nutrition and Physical Activity Guidelines for Cancer Survivors," *CA: A Cancer Journal for Clinicians* 62, no. 4 (July–August 2012): 243–74.

CHAPTER 8

NOURISH
YOUR BODY

H ippocrates advised, "Let food be your medicine and medicine be your food." Eating a healthy diet is one of the top three things that you can do to help yourself heal well. But wondering whether your diet caused your cancer—as some survivors do—will lead only to frustration. While having this information might be helpful, the truth is that you will never really know. Whenever I begin to dwell on what I might have done to avoid having cancer, I think of Ralph Waldo Emerson's advice: "Finish every day and be done with it. You have done what you could. Some blunders and absurdities no doubt crept in; forget them as soon as you can. . . . This day is all that is good and fair. It is too dear, with its hopes and invitations, to waste a moment on the yesterdays."

So, instead of spending a lot of energy wondering or worrying about the past, focus on what you can do *now* to improve your diet. What are you fueling your body with that can enhance healing and perhaps reduce your risk of having the cancer return? Usually people who eat really well can still make some dietary changes to improve their health— which is especially important during this period of recovery.

In 2001 my colleague Dr. Walter Willett, who is the chair of the Department of Nutrition at Harvard Medical School, published a groundbreaking book called *Eat, Drink, and Be Healthy*. In this book he charged that the U.S. Department of Agriculture's dietary recommendations, taught to children in grade school in the form of the food pyramid, were wrong: "At best, the USDA Pyramid offers wishy-washy, scientifically unfounded advice on an absolutely vital topic—what to eat. At worst, the misinformation contributes to overweight, poor health, and unnecessary early deaths."

Willett was clearly frustrated with the information that people were getting about how to eat. He gave the telling example of the "Great Nutrition Debate" sponsored in 2000 by the USDA, in which several authors of best-selling diet books discussed their philosophies. Willett described the event as a "mostly evidence-free food fight." He explained that "the wildly different recommendations presented in that three-hour session—eat lots of meat, don't eat any meat, eat lots of carbohydrates, don't eat any carbohydrates, cut your intake of fat to under 20 percent of calories, eat as much fat as you want, stay away from sugar, eat potatoes—neatly captured the chaos that we get in place of sound, sensible, and solid advice on healthy eating."

Following this debate, USDA undersecretary Shirley Watkins commented, "We will stand behind the Pyramid." However, Watkins was forced to eat her words in the face of tremendous pressure, including that from Willett's book, to change the food pyramid and make it more representative of what is known scientifically about healthy diets. Hence, Willet was instrumental in helping to improve the original food pyramid, and now the USDA is using a plate-shaped model to encourage healthy eating.

DIET AND CANCER

We know that diet is an extremely important component in cancer, and it is estimated that up to one-third or more of all cancers might be related to diet, exercise, and other lifestyle factors. Moreover, we have good evidence that optimal healing is hindered in people who are malnourished. A substantial amount of scientific evidence indicates that nutritionally optimizing survivors from diagnosis onward will help them to be stronger and healthier throughout treatment. Unfortunately, there is a great deal of misinformation in books, magazine articles, and on the Internet about cancer and nutrition; it is not always easy to sort out fact from fiction and what researchers surmise from what has been proved in scientific studies. For these reasons, it is worth taking a serious look at what you eat and how you can improve your nutritional status.

Food is important not only in preventing cancer (as well as other major causes of death and disability such as strokes and heart attacks) but also in healing. Foods contain carbohydrates, proteins, fats, vitamins, and minerals in varying amounts. The most significant of these for healing are proteins, complex substances that repair body tissue and maintain healthy immune responses. When there is not enough protein in the diet, recovery from illness and resistance to infection is hindered. Not surprisingly, protein supplementation prior to surgery may be helpful and is often part of prehabilitation protocols.

A great deal of research has been done on how nutritional status impacts wound healing. This research reveals that adequate nutrition is necessary for wound healing, avoiding infections, and, ultimately, patient survival. Good nutritional status also aids recovery in people who have sustained trauma and helps to heal the pressure sores that occur in the elderly and in people with poor skin sensation. Cancer patients who are malnourished may have a slower or incomplete recovery in terms of regaining strength and endurance. The place of diet in healing has been proven, and we can expect that continuing research will keep revealing more about how what we put into our bodies can affect our cells, both normal and malignant.

More than likely, you have already thought about nutrition and how it relates to the type of cancer you are dealing with. I am sure it is not news that cancer treatments, particularly chemotherapy, can wreak havoc on your appetite. Before, during, and sometimes after cancer treatment, many people should eat more protein than usual. Because of the effects of the treatment itself or its appetite-related side effects, however, you may not get enough of the nutrients you need. Most people have some fluctuation in their weight—either up or down—during treatment.

Because the food that we put in our mouths is something that we can *control* (in contrast with so many other things that we can't control), cancer survivors often place great importance on their diets. Although I want to underscore the value of a well-balanced diet that is high in fruits and vegetables, I think a pragmatic approach to nutrition is most beneficial—meaning that all most people need to do is to make a few minor changes in what they eat. I say this with one caveat—talk to your doctor or an oncology dietician about your nutritional needs, because he or she will be able to offer you specific advice that takes into account many factors such as your age, diagnosis, upcoming or current cancer treatment, other health problems, and so on.

Although I recommend taking a pragmatic approach to nutrition, after being diagnosed with cancer, it's easy to become a bit obsessed with this topic. I admit that I find myself worrying about how the food I eat will affect my body. I quickly squelch these thoughts and try to be practical and not obsessive. As I got ready to write this book, and for my own edification, I read all that I could about nutrition in the lay cancer literature. I found several books that advocated an extremely restrictive plant-based diet (essentially a vegan diet that contains no animal proteins). One woman wrote a thoughtful but not necessarily medically sound book called *Surviving Cancer*, in which she advocated "veggie overdosing" and stated, "Whereas I read that the average American eats seven pounds of broccoli a year, I eat seven pounds each *week*." Eating vegetables is important, but medical research does not currently support the theory of "veggie overdosing." A strict plant-based diet may in fact lack some vitamins, minerals, and complete proteins that are essential for good health.

Many books and articles that I read discussed the ill effects of the pesticides and hormones that are used to produce food. I must say that although I have a bachelor of science degree in food biochemistry, reading this material geared for the general public often made me feel anxious and overwhelmed. I frequently had the Bill Clinton "one wrong move" kind of feeling, which I know is *not* how diet works. Another response to some of what I read was, "Well, I need to just quit my job and devote myself to buying, preparing, and eating the most nutritious and chemical-free foods possible."

Other material that I read basically told me, "You've had cancer; be good to yourself and don't worry about what you eat." Obviously, these are the two extremes on the diet spectrum; perhaps each has some merit. But, as I began to write this book, I thought about what exactly I wanted readers to know about nutrition and cancer. Food is much more than what we put into our bodies. It is the focus around which we come together as a family, it is what we may turn to for comfort during periods of stress, and it is something that many of us thoroughly enjoy. What we eat may depend on cultural and religious values and traditions. I respect the fact that my readers come from all walks of life and there may be limits on the ways they can alter their diets. For all of us, though, this is what we need to focus on:

- What you eat can have a tremendous effect on your health—including cancer.
- When you are trying to heal from cancer or its treatments, a well-balanced diet is especially critical.
- One of the most important changes you can make in your diet is to try to eat five or more servings of fruits and vegetables daily, including a variety of colorful produce (the darker the color, the more nutrient dense the food).
- Be sure to get enough protein, but limit your consumption of meat and dairy products, especially those high in fat, and choose foods that help you maintain a healthy weight. Talk to your doctor or oncology dietician about whether you might benefit from protein supplementation prior to surgery or during other cancer treatments.
- Choose whole grains instead of processed foods and sugars.
- Organic foods are a wise choice, but sometimes they aren't available or they may be too expensive. If that's the case, it's better to eat the conventionally grown fruit and vegetables than to skip them altogether.
- Shop the perimeter of the grocery store where a lot of the healthier foods reside.
- Although this isn't always true, often the fewer the ingredients, the healthier the food (for example, an apple is healthier than sweetened apple sauce, which is healthier than apple pie).

Proteins

Adequate protein intake is essential during the healing process because proteins are the cell's primary building blocks. It is common for people undergoing chemotherapy, for instance, to significantly increase their dietary protein to facilitate healing, including the repair of damaged cells that are not cancerous and the regeneration of new cells. A rule of thumb for cancer survivors (whether in treatment or recently finished with therapy) is to multiply your weight by 0.5 and eat that many grams of protein. So, if you weigh 160 pounds, then you would eat 80 grams of protein each day. However, this amount may not be enough for some people, and it may be too much for others. The amount of protein that your doctor or dietitian recommends may depend on where you are in your treatment cycle and what type of therapy you are receiving. In terms of protein sources, plant-based proteins (for example, beans and nuts) have some advantages over animal proteins. Plant-based proteins provide phytochemicals (which are believed to help boost your immune system), vitamins, minerals, "good" fats, and fiber (fiber is found only in plant food).

Fruits and Vegetables

Eating at least five servings each day of fruits and vegetables is one of the best things you can do for your body. Many substances found in this food group help with healing and may help reduce the risk of cancer recurrence. For example, broccoli and other cruciferous vegetables (see Table 8.1) contain compounds that may reduce the risk of some types of cancer, such as breast, colon, and bladder cancer. These compounds are called *phytochemicals* and are believed to have antitumor effects. Phytochemicals (chemicals produced by plants) are also found in beans, grains, and other foods. Some of the more commonly known phytochemicals include ascorbic and folic acid, beta-carotene, and vitamin E.

Fruits and vegetables are also good sources of antioxidants (a subcategory of phytochemicals), which are believed to lower cancer risk. Antioxidants such as vitamins C and E, beta-carotene, and lycopene are found in many fruits and vegetables. Lycopene, believed to be a par-

Table 8.1. Examples of Cruciferous Vegetables

Cruciferous vegetables are so named because they are plants that have four flowers in a cluster, resembling a cross.

Arugula	Kale
Bok choy	Mustard greens
Broccoli	Radishes
Brussels sprouts	Rutabagas
Cauliflower	Turnips
Collard greens	Watercress

ticularly powerful antioxidant, is found in tomatoes, apricots, guavas, watermelons, papayas, and pink grapefruit. As a rule, darker-colored fruits and vegetables are rich in phytochemicals and antioxidants.

Other substances that are present in these foods also help with healing and may reduce the risk of cancer. These substances include carotenoids (present in orange-colored foods such as carrots, yams, apricots, and cantaloupes), anthocyanins (in tomatoes, red peppers, and pink grapefruit juice), and sulfides (in garlic and onions). It is believed that fruits and vegetables contain still more specific chemicals—not yet identified—that aid in cancer healing or prevention.

In some studies, fruit and vegetable supplements in pill form have been shown to raise antioxidant levels in the blood. The primary concern with such supplements is that while we know that fruits and vegetables are important in helping to reduce the risk of certain kinds of cancer, we aren't sure precisely which ingredients are the most important. In addition, since these foods contain possibly helpful components that have not been identified yet, the pill supplements are almost certainly not as good as eating at least five servings daily of fruits and vegetables. I generally recommend that people take a single multivitamin daily and only suggest additional supplements in some instances when it is clear that they are not consuming fruits and vegetables and are unable to change their diet to include at least some of these foods.

Nutritional supplements that contain megadoses of vitamins or antioxidants are not recommended. Whether people with cancer should take supplements that contain antioxidants is a topic of much debate in the oncology community. Although increasing the phytochemicals in your diet is an excellent idea, taking supplements might be "too much of a good thing." For example, many of the chemotherapeutic agents work via pathways that may be adversely affected by antioxidants. This means that the prescribed medications may not be as effective. The concept of "oxidative stress," which has not been fully explored, could mean that taking too many antioxidants might depress rather than enhance one's immune system. If you are actively in treatment, my advice on antioxidants is to talk to your oncologist. If you have finished treatment, it may be worthwhile to take a small dose but avoid megadoses.

Carbohydrates

Carbohydrates can be classified as complex (vegetables, nuts, seeds, legumes, and whole grains) and simple (bread, pasta, and other starches). Sugars such as table sugar, honey, and sweets are sometimes considered a third category. When they are digested, all carbohydrates are broken down into sugar, which enters the bloodstream and prompts the pancreas to respond by releasing insulin to lower the blood sugar level. The *glycemic index*—which is a method of measuring how fast and how high a person's blood sugar level rises—is based on this process. *Your goal should be to eat foods with a low glycemic level because they don't cause rapid or extreme fluctuations in blood sugar levels.* Complex carbohydrates are among the foods that serve this purpose.

Complex carbohydrate sources (listed in Table 8.2) include whole grains, which differ from refined grains in that they contain the germ (sprout of a new plant), the endosperm (the seed's source of energy), and the bran (the outer layer). Refined grains (for example, white flour) have had the bran and the germ—which contain important nutrients—removed during the milling process. The nutrients that are lost may include B vitamins, iron, zinc, phytochemicals, vitamin E, and fiber. Moreover, milling the grain means that it is digested more quickly and therefore causes the blood sugar to rise fast and high.

Table 8.2. Sources of Complex Carbohydrates	
Arborio rice	Fresh fruits
Barley	Fresh vegetables
Basmati	Kasha
Black, fava, kidney, lima, mung,	Millet
navy, pinto, and white beans*	Oats
Bran	Rye
Brown and wild rice	Whole-grain breakfast cereal
Bulgur	(100% whole grain)
Chickpeas	Whole wheat
Flaxseed	

*Beans have the added benefit of being high in protein.

Fats

Fats have a bad reputation that is in large part deserved. Some fat in the diet is needed, though. For cancer survivors who are underweight, dietary fat recommendations may be higher than normal. But for most people it is best to stick to small amounts of polyunsaturated and mono-unsaturated fats, which are considered "good fats." Saturated fats (as in whole milk and high-fat meats) and trans fats (as in margarine, vegetable shortening, and packaged breads, cakes, cookies, and crackers) are "bad fats." You should eat these foods in very limited quantities or avoid them completely. Vegetable oils (for example, grape seed, corn, olive, and canola), nuts, and some fish (for example, salmon, lake trout, tuna, and herring) are sources of "good fats."

How you cook your food can also influence the fat content. Try to use only extra-virgin olive oil or canola oil to cook. Braising, pan searing, roasting, and stewing are all cooking methods that help keep fat levels low. Limit your consumption of grilled or blackened meat, poultry, and fish because of the potential for production of polycyclic aromatic hydrocarbons, which are thought to be *carcinogens* (cancer-causing substances). If you really enjoy grilled food, marinate or partially cook the meat before grilling so that you can reduce the grilling time. Nitrates used in cured meats (bacon, sausage, and smoked meats) may also be carcinogens.

Vitamin and Mineral Supplements

A daily multivitamin can help to ensure that you are receiving the vitamins you need. Not everyone needs to take a multivitamin, but most people can benefit from taking one as a sort of "insurance policy." For those who are anemic because of an iron deficiency, this practice can be helpful as well, since multivitamin supplements usually also contain iron. Iron can contribute to constipation, however; so if you are not deficient in iron and you are concerned about constipation, choose one of the low-iron multivitamins (often labeled as a geriatric alternative). Pick one that does not exceed 100 percent of the USRDA (recommended daily allowance). There is no difference between natural and synthetic products.

Protecting your bones is extremely important. Fractures are a serious and common cause of disability in people who have either mild bone loss (osteopenia) or more severe bone loss (osteoporosis). Osteoporosis has been studied especially in postmenopausal women, but anyone (including young men who normally have strong bones) who has been through cancer treatment may be at risk for decreased bone mineral density. Simple imaging studies (usually specialized x-rays) are a good way to determine whether you have osteopenia or osteoporosis. Ask your doctor whether you are at risk for bone loss due to your cancer treatments or perhaps factors such as other medical problems or your age. Either your primary care doctor or your oncologist can order bone mineral density studies.

Treatment for bone loss varies depending on the extent of the loss and other factors. Although specific treatment recommendations are beyond the scope of this discussion, it is reasonable for most people to follow the guidelines established by the National Osteoporosis Foundation, which are summarized in Table 8.3. While you are receiving chemotherapy or other treatment, your doctor or registered dietitian may recommend different doses (usually a little higher) from those in Table 8.3. There may also be medical conditions, such as a recent or severe history of kidney stones (which could be exacerbated by calcium supplements) or a history of skin cancer (which keeps you out of the sun and reduces your ability to get vitamin D), that influence your

Table 8.3. Calcium and Vitamin D Guidelines for Osteoporosis Prevention in Women

Calcium
At least 1,200 mg per day (1,000 mg per day for women under 50), including supplements if necessary. (American women typically consume about 600 mg of calcium per day in their diets, leaving a deficit of 600 mg, which a supplement can cover.)

Vitamin D
400 to 800 IU per day for individuals at risk of deficiency.

Recommended Supplements: There are many supplements to choose from. Calcium citrate (Citracal) and calcium carbonate (Tums and Viactiv) are the forms of calcium that are best absorbed by the body. It is recommended that the supplements be taken in the afternoon or evening, with food, and only 500 mg at one time (roughly the amount contained in one pill).

Source: Guidelines provided by the National Osteoporosis Foundation, nof.org.

doctor's recommendation regarding calcium or vitamin D supplements. Recognize, too, that regular weight-bearing exercise helps to promote stronger bones and that caffeine, alcohol, and tobacco can all have a negative impact on bone density.

WHY CHOOSE ORGANIC FOODS?

We don't know much about the long-term effects of the added chemicals that are commonly used to grow or preserve food. We will probably learn eventually that such things as bovine growth hormone and irradiated or genetically engineered food are either not particularly harmful or that they can contribute to tumor growth. *It is unlikely that we'll find out that these things are good for our health.* Therefore, when people ask me whether they should eat organic food, I answer that it is wise to incorporate certified organic food into your diet as much as possible. Only produce labeled "organic" is certified as meeting USDA organic standards. "Natural" does not mean organic.

Certified organic food, though sometimes more expensive than nonorganic food, is grown with a number of restrictions. For example, organic farmers in the meat industry give no antibiotics or growth hormones to their animals. Organic food also is grown and marketed without conventional pesticides, fertilizers, or ionizing radiation. The National Organic Program is a federal law that requires all organic food products to meet the same standards and be certified under the same certification process. Along with this program, the USDA has developed strict labeling rules to help consumers know the specific content of the organic food they buy. The USDA organic seal means that at least 95 percent of the product is organic.

If organic foods are not an option, then be sure to wash fruits and vegetables thoroughly under clean, cold, running water before eating them. Wash thoroughly even if the produce will be cooked, peeled, or cut. Avoid using rinses, soaps, or chlorine bleach solutions.

A HEALING DIET

If you are confused about what is a healthy diet, you are not alone. There are numerous theories, many of which seem quite plausible, about what and how much to eat. My goal is to present a reasonable approach for most cancer survivors. If you have unique issues relating to your health status or your cultural, religious, or other beliefs, you may benefit from talking to your doctor or to a registered dietitian who specializes in oncology (see the next section, "Advice from the Experts"). Individuals who need to gain or lose weight, who are diabetic, or who have other health issues requiring diet modifications may especially need a professional consultation. It will also be helpful for people such as vegans who follow fairly strict dietary regimens. Keep in mind that while you may know a lot about nutrition, your doctor or dietitian may be able to contribute some useful pearls that are specific to your particular circumstances.

In Willett's excellent book on nutrition, he tells people that there is "no single healthy diet." Rather, there are some basic rules of good nutrition. You should eat what you enjoy eating (focusing on the foods you like that follow the basic rules of good nutrition), eat what your family eats, and eat foods that are part of the cultural tradition in which you feel most comfortable. Dr. Willett also constructs his own food pyramid, which he calls the Healthy Eating Pyramid. He recommends the following:

- Eat red meat, butter, white rice and bread, potatoes, pasta, and sweets sparingly.
- Eat dairy foods or take calcium supplements one to two times a day.
- Eat fish, poultry, and eggs zero to two times a day.
- Eat nuts and legumes one to three times a day.
- Eat vegetables in abundance.
- Eat fruits two to three times a day.
- Eat whole grains at most meals.
- Use plant oils such as olive, canola, soy, corn, sunflower, and peanut.

These are general guidelines, and they don't necessarily take into account the fact that a person undergoing cell repair may need more protein. Your doctor or dietitian can guide you in any specifics that might pertain to your recovery.

My dietary suggestions to help a person heal from cancer and its treatment are summarized as follows:

1. Eat five or more servings of fruits and vegetables daily—choosing a variety of colorful produce.
2. Talk to your doctor or dietitian about how much protein you need to heal well.
3. Eat certified organic foods when possible.
4. Choose whole grains instead of processed grains and flours.
5. Limit the amount of refined sugar you eat, and choose nutrient-dense foods instead.
6. Eat a diet low in fat, but do not eliminate fat altogether.
7. Avoid nicotine completely and alcohol as much as possible.
8. Be sure to get enough calcium (1,000–1,200 mg daily) and vitamin D (200–600 IU daily).
9. Consider taking a daily multivitamin that does not exceed 100 percent of the USRDA.
10. Talk to your doctor about any supplements you are taking or thinking of starting.

Eating a nutritious diet is one of the three most important healing measures that are under your control. A now-famous example of how diet affects health adversely comes from Morgan Spurlock's documentary *Super Size Me*. As you may recall, Spurlock decided to eat at McDonald's for every meal for one month. The *Washington Post* reported the effect of this diet on his health: "At the end of his experiment the once-healthy Spurlock waddled out of the last McDonald's with a splotchy face, a reduced libido and 25 extra pounds. He had been transformed into a pudgy young man with dangerously high cholesterol, chest pains and a liver that was overwhelmed by the fat in his system." This is an extreme case, and Spurlock obviously undertook his experiment to make a point: a healthy diet is important for everyone.

ADVICE FROM THE EXPERTS

At any juncture in your treatment or recovery, it is a wise idea to check in with a registered dietitian who specializes in oncology. She or he can offer invaluable tips based on your diagnosis, the treatment you have undergone, your current diet and weight, and other factors that are individual to you. Many people without any legitimate training or credentials offer nutrition advice. When seeking advice from a professional, you need to ask whether the person is a registered dietitian (RD), a licensed dietitian (LD or LDN), or both. Registered and licensed dietitians have completed required coursework, passed a professional qualifying examination, and maintain registration via regular yearly studies verified by the American Dietetic Association and the state they live in. Other good sources of information on diet and nutrition are the National Cancer Institute and the National Center for Complementary and Alternative Medicine, which are both listed in the appendix. The book *Eating Well, Staying Well During and After Cancer* is a terrific resource published by the American Cancer Society.

What about Soy?

Eating soy, which contains a subgroup of phytochemicals called *flavonoids*, is controversial, because some components of flavonoids resemble estrogen. Estrogen is a factor in some hormonally driven tumors, and it is possible that soy might help some tumors to thrive. We don't understand this matter well, but as a precaution I advise my patients to avoid soy if they have an estrogen-receptor-positive tumor. If you are not sure what to do, ask your doctor about soy and other foods that contain flavonoids (for example, garbanzo beans, chickpeas, licorice, and tea).

Nicotine

We all know that smoking is bad for our health, but nicotine is very addictive and its hold can be strong. The nicotine in chewing tobacco and snuff is also a potential toxin. Despite the well-known ill effects of nicotine, we live in a world where its use is glamorized—perhaps nowhere more so than in the movies. Joe Eszterhas is a successful Hollywood screenwriter who admits that he deliberately glamorized smoking in his movies. In his more-than-seven-hundred-page tome, *Hollywood Animal*, he reveals a dark side of the movie industry. There he comments on the success of one of his movies: "After the worldwide success of *Basic Instinct*, a tobacco company released Basic cigarettes, no doubt inspired by the sex/smoking scenes in the movie. Thanks to me, even more people in the world would be smoking." Later, Eszterhas developed laryngeal cancer and began to advocate against showing actors smoking.

Most people who smoke begin in their youth when they are particularly vulnerable, least knowledgeable, and years away from the negative effects that nicotine can have on their health. Many cancer survivors feel guilty about smoking currently or having smoked in the past. When I talk to my patients about smoking, I always tread lightly. I know that they beat themselves up over this issue, and the last thing I want to do is to cause them more distress. Medical literature reveals, however, that patients often have the most success quitting when their doctor plays an active role in helping to motivate them.

If you have smoked in the past but have now stopped, you are doing something very beneficial for your health. Your body is powerful in ridding itself of toxins and recovering. If you have had one of the types of cancer that is linked with smoking, the treatment you underwent and your body's own healing mechanisms can make an enormous difference. So, my advice is to focus on your success as much as possible. Quitting smoking can be very difficult and you should be congratulated for doing it. Use that success to help you to improve other health habits as well.

If you smoke now and want to quit, you may be one of the people who have tried in the past to quit, without lasting success. Rather than considering your previous attempts as failures, keep in mind that the road to success is typically a process that includes short or long periods (perhaps a day, a month, or a year) without smoking. The same is true of discontinuing the use of chewing tobacco and snuff. Therefore, if you have stopped smoking even for a short time in the past, you have achieved some success. Moreover, right now is probably a time in your life when you are extremely motivated to quit. Increased motivation, along with your past short-term successes, can be the key to stopping forever. I advise my patients to consider these reasons for not smoking:

- Nicotine is toxic to your body and can cause cancer.
- Smoking reduces your ability to physically heal (many surgeons won't do surgery on people who smoke, because of the increased risk of pulmonary complications and wound infections).

I ask my patients to have a frank discussion with their primary care physicians about how they can stop smoking. Also consider the sage stop-smoking advice that Ann Landers gave millions of Americans:

- Make the decision to quit. Set yourself a quit date and prepare yourself for the transition.
- Become aware of your pattern of use, identifying trigger places, people, and activities.
- Explore on paper your motivations for quitting. Carry a list with you of your top three reasons.
- Start an exercise program.
- Set up a social support system.
- Commit to doing what it takes to get through the short-term discomfort.
- Smoke your last cigarette and say good-bye.

- Dispose of all tobacco products and paraphernalia (with the exceptions of nicotine gum or patches if you are using one of these methods to help you stop smoking).
- Drink lots of water to help eliminate nicotine from your system.
- Take deep breaths to keep you centered.
- Take action whenever an urge presents itself. Call your support people. Pray. Take a walk. Stretch. The urge *will* pass.
- Envision yourself already smoke-free.
- Modify your lifestyle to support your smoke-free status.
- Change your daily routines to avoid old triggers.
- Develop a system of rewards for yourself.
- Develop new interests to give your life a positive focus, and redirect your energy.

The American Cancer Society (ACS) recommends that you stop smoking "cold turkey." Some people can gradually wean themselves off cigarettes, but more people successfully quit when they stop abruptly. For a good and quick reference guide on how to quit smoking, check out the book *Kicking Butts* (available from the ACS).

Alcohol

Alcohol has often been misrepresented by the media as potentially having important protective and restorative health advantages. The truth is that we have a *little* bit of research that suggests that alcohol—in unknown but probably quite small quantities—*may* be somewhat helpful in preventing heart diseases. We have a much, much greater body of research showing that alcohol is a toxic substance and can be harmful to some people who drink moderately. Alcohol has been linked to a number of serious medical conditions, including dementia, liver cirrhosis, heart disease, and cancer. Some of the cancers in which alcohol may play a role include cancers of the breast, the liver, the pancreas, the mouth, the throat, the esophagus, the colon, and the rectum. Alcohol also can slow physical healing by damaging cells and can make recovery more difficult. For example, one side effect of some chemotherapeutic drugs is neuropathy: the medications injure nerve cells, usually in the hands and feet. The condition can improve over time as your body heals;

however, alcohol (in significant quantities) may also cause neuropathy. Therefore, people with neuropathy might not heal as well if they drink excessively.

Some people might be surprised at the relatively small amounts of alcohol that have been linked with different types of cancer. For instance, more than fifty studies have been done over the past ten years looking at the relationship between breast cancer and alcohol. In a recent study, researcher Anette Lykke Petri and her colleagues concluded, "Among postmenopausal women, spirits of more than six drinks per week increases breast cancer risk."

If you have had cancer, you might want to consider having an alcoholic beverage or two only on rare social occasions or abstaining altogether. It is the regular, daily or almost daily, consumption of alcohol that seems to put people at the greatest risk for its toxic effects. If you enjoy having a drink or two or even a few drinks at night, think about how important this routine is to you. I always ask my patients, "Do you think you might be using alcohol in a medicinal way to help control stress or your mood?"

When actor Michael J. Fox was diagnosed with early-onset Parkinson's disease, he spent the next few years recklessly, in terms of caring for himself physically and emotionally. He wrote a book about his experiences called *Lucky Man*, in which he shares the hold alcohol had over him: "I craved alcohol as a direct response to the need I felt to escape my situation. Joyless and secretive, I drank to disassociate; drinking now was about isolation and self-medication." Later, after he had stopped drinking and reconnected with his loved ones, he reflected on his life: "Nobody would ever choose to have this [illness] visited upon them. Still, this unexpected crisis forced a fundamental life decision: adopt a siege mentality—or embark upon a journey. Whatever it was— courage? Acceptance? Wisdom?—that finally allowed me to go down the second road (after spending a few disastrous years on the first) was unquestionably a gift—and absent this neurophysiological catastrophe, I would never have opened it, or been so profoundly enriched. That's why I consider myself a lucky man."

When my patients tell me that they are using alcohol to self-medicate, I talk about the healthier alternatives that can be used to improve one's mood and stress level. I also tell patients that alcohol is a depressant: while they might initially feel a bit less stressed, over time their mood will usually not improve but will deteriorate. Many people don't recognize this important fact. For more information on how mood may affect physical healing and cancer recurrence, see chapter 11.

If you drink regularly, regardless of the quantity, consider taking a three-month break. During that time, establish new habits to reduce stress, such as meditation or exercise. If you are concerned about taking three months off from drinking, talk to your doctor about the reasons for your concern. She or he should be able to help you achieve this goal.

Obviously, alcohol means different things to people. For some it is part of sacred religious traditions. For others it is associated with having a good time at a party. Still others value alcohol as part of their daily routine. Of course, alcohol can also be a very negative force in someone's life—especially if taken in excessive quantities. If you have had cancer and you are trying to physically heal, the main questions you should be asking are, "Might alcohol adversely affect my health? And, if so, am I able to reduce the amount that I consume, or abstain altogether?"

FIGHTING FATIGUE WITH FOOD

Fatigue is a common problem in people who are undergoing cancer treatment or have finished with therapy and are in the process of healing. Although a person's diet may be just one factor among the many reasons for fatigue, in some people diet plays a significant role. So, what can you do diet-wise to have more energy and endurance? Consider the following suggestions:

- Be sure you are getting enough protein in your diet. Talk to your doctor and your dietitian about your protein needs. It may help to keep a log for a week or two in which you record how much protein you are consuming. Then, as a trial at home, increase the amount for a couple of weeks and see whether you feel a bit more energetic.
- Don't skip any meals, especially breakfast. Three nutritious meals each day are essential for getting enough nutrients to heal well and feel good. Don't skip (or skimp on) meals.

- Try eating three medium-sized meals with two nutritious snacks in between. Sometimes people have difficulty maintaining their blood sugar levels between meals, and eating a healthy snack can be just the boost they need to have more energy.
- Avoid refined sugar and simple carbohydrates (sweets, crackers, chips, etc.). These tend to give you a quick energy boost by increasing your blood sugar to a fairly high level. Your body immediately responds by releasing insulin to reduce the level of blood sugar, which drops precipitously, making you feel sluggish and tired.
- Take in adequate calories. On average, people should eat about 15 calories for each pound they weigh in order to maintain their weight. If you want to gain weight, you'll need to eat additional calories (around 500 extra calories per day is a reasonable number to shoot for). If you want to lose weight, eat fewer calories. However, if you don't consume enough calories to keep your energy level up, you'll feel lousy while you lose weight. Weight loss needs to be gradual, so that your energy level will be optimal.
- Iron has long been believed to be a panacea for illness and a great protector of good health. The practice of using iron medicinally came to America with European immigrants. It wasn't until 1938 that a requirement of "therapeutic value" for drugs was instituted; and so prior to this date, with no proven efficacy, iron was used in many tonics and elixirs. Overdoses were not uncommon and could cause problems including severe constipation, blackening of the teeth, and even death. Today we know that iron has very limited uses, and doctors usually prescribe it only for people who have a certain type of blood anemia. Some people treated for cancer will be deficient in iron and may need to take a supplement. Check with your doctor, though, before taking an iron supplement.
- Stay well hydrated. The best drinks are water, fruit and vegetable juices, and milk. It is best to avoid or limit your intake of caffeinated drinks (including coffee and tea), sodas, and alcohol. Some cancer survivors like to drink green tea, which may or may not be helpful (it is a controversial issue). If you drink green tea, you should have other sources of hydration as well.

Special Dietary Concerns in Cancer Survivors

There are many, many issues that may play a role in the nutritional state of a cancer survivor. The treatments may cause an increase or decrease in appetite. Nausea, vomiting, diarrhea, or constipation may be present. Intestinal surgery or removal of vital organs such as the pancreas can significantly impact one's diet and nutritional status. These problems need to be addressed individually based on the person's diagnosis, treatment, current weight, nutritional status, and other issues such as ongoing fatigue or nausea. If you have concerns about your diet or related matters, talk to your doctor and consider consulting a dietitian.

References

W. C. Willett, *Eat, Drink, and Be Healthy* (New York: Simon and Schuster, 2001), pp. 13, 17.

M. Levine, *Surviving Cancer* (New York: Broadway Books, 2001), p. 142.

R. Givhan, "Lord of the Fries: Morgan Spurlock Got His Fill of Ailments Making 'Super Size Me,' but He's Been Fortified by Its Impact," *Washington Post*, May 2, 2004, p. N1.

J. Eszterhas, *Hollywood Animal* (New York: Random House, 2004), p. 8.

A. Landers, "Keys to Living Smoke-Free," *Buffalo (New York) News*, January 2, 1999, final ed., p. A7.

A. S. Brittain, ed., *Kicking Butts: Quit Smoking and Take Charge of Your Health* (Atlanta, GA: American Cancer Society, 2003).

A. L. Petri, A. Tjonneland, M. Gamborg, D. Johansen, S. Hoidrup, T. I. A. Sorensen, and M. Gronbaek, "Alcohol Intake, Type of Beverage, and Risk of Breast Cancer in Pre- and Postmenopausal Women," *Alcoholism: Clinical and Experimental Research* 28 (2004): 1084.

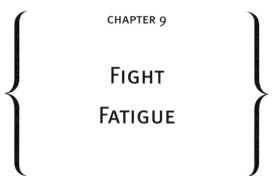

CHAPTER 9

FIGHT

FATIGUE

Fatigue is the most common complaint among cancer survivors, and it may impact every facet of their daily lives. Fatigue often occurs with other symptoms, such as pain and anxiety. When they occur together, they are called *cluster symptoms*. Although it is important to address all of the symptoms that occur in the cluster, frequently there is a *sentinel symptom* that is the main problem. For example, let's say that a woman just finished treatment for breast cancer and she has an issue with the rotator cuff in her shoulder. While she is sleeping, she may have pain that awakens her. It would be normal for her to be worried about this pain—thinking that perhaps her cancer has returned. So, now in addition to having pain, she's a bit anxious and also not sleeping well, so she's fatigued. Her shoulder pain is the sentinel symptom, and treating this symptom will likely improve all of her cluster symptoms.

Patients and healthcare professionals often have different perceptions about fatigue. Healthcare professionals frequently underestimate its frequency, severity, and impact on quality of life. But many patients report that fatigue is a more debilitating symptom than pain—often citing it as a major life concern and not just a bothersome side effect. Patients notoriously underreport fatigue to their doctors, though, either by not mentioning it at all or by failing to explain clearly the impact fatigue is having on their ability to function. One reason for this lack of communication might be a belief by both patients and healthcare professionals that tiredness is just something to be endured rather than a real symptom. Of course, it is also true that, in the presence of a life-threatening illness, everyone's focus is on saving the sick person's life.

Nevertheless, chronic fatigue can certainly have a negative impact on one's ability to heal. For example, a person who is tired is less likely to be physically active, and inactivity leads to reduced stamina and becoming yet more physically unfit. In addition, fatigue might play a role in the prognosis of a cancer patient—a topic I'll address later in this chapter. Thus, the fullest recovery may depend on identifying and addressing symptoms of fatigue.

Cancer-Related Fatigue

According to guidelines published by the National Comprehensive Cancer Network, cancer-related fatigue is defined as a "distressing, persistent, subjective sense of tiredness or exhaustion related to cancer or cancer treatment that is not proportional to recent activity and interferes with usual functioning." This type of fatigue is often described as an overwhelming tiredness that is not relieved by rest. Normal fatigue occurs at the end of a long and busy day and is usually not overwhelming. Normal weariness is predictable and not intense. The National Comprehensive Cancer Network lists a number of factors that are likely to contribute to fatigue in cancer patients: pain, depression and anxiety, inactivity, sleep problems, poor nutrition, medications, and other health conditions. The tumor itself may also be a factor. Thus, cancer-related fatigue is most likely caused by a combination of factors. Fatigue is a symptom that plagued me and was by far the most debilitating symptom during my recovery.

How does cancer cause fatigue? There are many theories. Tumor cells compete for nutrients, often at the expense of the normal cells' growth. The cancer literature sometimes suggests that the resulting fatigue is related to the direct effect of cancer and the "tumor burden." This type of fatigue is almost certainly influenced at least in part by the type of cancer and the stage of disease, although these relationships have not been thoroughly sorted out. Researchers have also found that fatigue may predate the diagnosis of cancer, further indicating that the growth of the cancer itself may be responsible.

Fatigue may be a side effect of cancer treatment—a problem that we don't fully understand. We do know that the type of therapy, the dose and length of a particular treatment, and whether it is combined with other interventions are factors that influence fatigue. The goal of cancer treatment is to kill malignant cells. Unfortunately, most therapies damage healthy cells as well. One theory of cancer-related fatigue as it relates directly to treatment is that your body becomes tired from working so hard to repair the damage to healthy cells and tissues. Other theories focus on how the chemotherapy or other treatments may affect normal biochemical reactions in the body. And there are more theories that suggest other potential factors in cancer-related fatigue (see Table 9.1).

We do know that cancer-related fatigue can last for weeks, months, or even years following treatment. The type of cancer may be a factor as well as the treatment regimen. Nearly every oncology treatment, including biological therapy (for example, interferon and interleukin-2), chemotherapy, radiation, and bone marrow transplants, has been associated with significant fatigue that may be prolonged. Cancer-related fatigue also seems to be cumulative. For example, people who are undergoing radiation treatment seem to experience more severe tiredness later in the course than near the beginning. Researchers are studying

---

Table 9.1. Factors Contributing to Cancer-Related Fatigue

Direct effect of the tumor

Destruction of normal cells along with cancer cells by treatment (repairing the damage to healthy cells and tissues may cause fatigue)

Decreased nutrition resulting from the side effects of treatments (nausea, mouth sores, taste changes, diarrhea, heartburn)

Infections

Hormonal imbalances

Reduction in blood counts by chemotherapy (anemia may occur as a result)

Effects of medicines used to treat the cancer or alleviate side effects

Chronic pain

Stress

Anxiety or depression

Lack of sleep or poor sleep

Lack of exercise/deconditioning

who is at the highest risk for this troubling symptom, and not surprisingly it seems to be worse for individuals on active treatment or those who have received a combination of treatments. In a recent study of more than two thousand cancer survivors that was published in the journal *Cancer*, researchers found that moderate to severe fatigue was reported by 45 percent of the patients who were receiving active treatment and 29 percent of survivors who had completed their treatment and had no evidence of active cancer (they were cured or in remission). In people currently undergoing treatment, fatigue was more profound in those who were taking strong opioid medications for pain, had lost more than 5 percent of their body weight within the past six months, had a history of depression or were taking ten or more medications. Survivors who were not on active treatment were more likely to be fatigued if they were struggling with physical performance and activity or had a history of depression.

If you have several of these symptoms most of the days of the week, then cancer-related fatigue might be the culprit:

Decreased motivation to engage in your usual activities
Difficulty falling asleep or staying asleep, or sleeping more than usual
Waking up and feeling that sleep didn't refresh you
Struggling to be more active
Feeling frustrated, sad, or irritable about being tired
Difficulty in completing your daily tasks due to fatigue
Problems with your ability to concentrate or with your short-term memory
Feeling exhausted for several hours after physically exerting yourself
Having your legs or arms feel heavy

To treat cancer-related fatigue, your healthcare provider must ascertain that fatigue is affecting you socially, occupationally, or in other important areas of daily activity. He or she will also want to rule out contributing factors such as major depression, general lack of fitness, and anemia. Cancer survivors may, of course, have fatigue that is unrelated to the cancer diagnosis or its treatment, and there is some crossover between general fatigue and cancer-related fatigue. For example, anemia can be a side effect of cancer treatment, or it may be related to another issue such as not consuming enough iron. See Table 9.2 for causes of fatigue not necessarily related to cancer.

You may already have a good idea of whether fatigue is affecting your ability to heal. If you aren't sure, try answering the questions listed in Table 9.3. These are questions that I often ask my patients. If you answer yes to two or more, it is likely that your lack of energy is having

Table 9.2. Causes of Fatigue in the General Population	
Anemia	Hypothyroidism or other hormonal
Anxiety	imbalances
Chronic illnesses (diabetes,	Illicit drug or alcohol dependency
rheumatoid arthritis, etc.)	Overdose or side effects of
Chronic fatigue syndrome	prescribed medication
Chronic infection	Postoperative deconditioning
Chronic pain	Postpolio syndrome
Depression	Postviral infection
Excessive exercise or muscular	Respiratory disorders (asthma,
overexertion	emphysema, etc.)
Fibromyalgia	Sleep disorders (insomnia, sleep
Heart disease	apnea, etc.)
Hypoglycemia (low blood sugar)	

Table 9.3. Assessing Fatigue

1. Do you feel tired when you awaken in the morning?
2. Do you have a sense of overwhelming fatigue despite sleeping well?
3. Is sleep nonrestorative for you?
4. Are you a restless sleeper?
5. Do you have difficulty falling asleep or falling back to sleep?
6. Do you snore?
7. Do you rest or nap during the day?
8. Have you curtailed or modified your activities because of a reduced energy level?
9. Is fatigue affecting your home life, work, or recreation?
10. Do you have difficulty with memory, concentration, attention, or finding words?
11. Is your energy level different now than it was before you were diagnosed and treated for cancer? If so, in what ways?

an impact and that you could benefit from some intervention. Your yes answers do not mean that the fatigue you are experiencing is cancer related, but they do indicate that you should consider seeking assistance from your doctor to define the cause of your fatigue and discover the available treatment options.

A Good Night's Rest

Religious texts dating back to antiquity contain references to the healing powers of sleep. The importance of sleep has been well understood. Scholar Sonia Ancoli-Israel has written about the Hebrew view of sleep as a medicine:

> [Our ancestors] referred to the function of sleep as being restorative. They deplored sleep deprivation, believing that it impaired life. They felt that excessive sleepiness was harmful. They understood that insomnia could be caused by stress and anxiety and by excessive alcohol, and that physical activity (exercise) and drinking milk could improve sleep. . . . Although we think we have discovered many new features about sleep disorders, most of what we do is to match scientific data to ideas documented in the Bible and the Talmud. Our modern scientific knowledge about sleep is not new and existed even in biblical times. . . . The conclusion for then and now is that "sleep is not tangible" (Talmud Shevu'oth 25a), that is, although the rabbis may not have fully understood sleep, they left enough clues and interpretations that agree with what science has verified thousands of years later.

The importance of a good night's rest should never be underestimated—though it often is. Poor sleep leading to fatigue is a major problem in cancer survivors, and yet it is frequently overlooked by both patients and their doctors. Although we know that our ancestors have long realized the importance of sleep, within the medical community it is only recently that we have intensely studied the effect of sleep on health and disease.

There is much left to be discovered, but we now know that the immune system and the sleep-wake cycle share a number of important chemical compounds. For example, a lack of sleep is associated in part with an increase in norepinephrine levels and decreased activity of natural killer cells, which are important in the immune response to cancer. Other immune factors that have been reported to have significant effects on sleep include interleukin-1, tumor necrosis factor-alpha, and interferon. Significant detrimental effects on immune functioning can be seen after a few days of total sleep deprivation or after several days of partial sleep deprivation.

Insufficient sleep is also associated with a reduction in the level of melatonin—a hormone produced by the pineal gland in the brain that is known to have antioxidant properties and affect immune function. In addition, melatonin has been linked to the regulation of circadian and seasonal rhythms, the health of the retina in the eye, and stopping or slowing tumor growth. It is thought that this hormone may affect cancer through its ability to act as a free-radical scavenger and an antioxidant. Because melatonin levels peak at night while a person sleeps, the absence of sleep or poor sleep may significantly influence melatonin release. In a review article on this topic, Russel Reiter noted that "interactions between melatonin and the immune system have been known for roughly 30 years, and in virtually all cases, melatonin has been proven to have immunoenhancing effects. . . . A considerable amount of evidence has been amassed which documents the efficacy of melatonin in reducing tumour growth. While the bulk of these data have accrued from studies on experimental animals, trials in humans with a wide variety of different cancers are also suggestive of the onco-static [tumor-inhibiting] actions of melatonin." It is not known whether taking melatonin as a "natural" product will have the same positive effect as the melatonin your body produces. Melatonin can be obtained from beef cattle or it can be chemically synthesized. Be aware, however, that the melatonin supplements in a health food store can vary widely from brand to brand in both dose and ingredients.

As a recent review titled "Update on the Role of Melatonin in the Prevention of Cancer Tumorigenesis and the Management of Cancer Correlates, Such as Sleep-Wake and Mood Disturbances" reports, there have been many conflicting studies about how melatonin may impact the growth of cancer cells, but it is generally believed to have a positive influence in protecting your immune system. Of course, it makes sense that improving your sleep will be helpful to you in many ways. Normal sleep involves two distinct types of sleep: non-rapid-eye-movement (NREM) sleep and rapid-eye-movement (REM) sleep. A period of sleep begins with the NREM type and progresses to REM sleep, which is the active phase of sleep, during which dreams occur. Inadequate sleep can result from various factors, including too little rest in general, inadequate REM sleep, frequent arousals, difficulty falling asleep, lack of sufficient oxygen during sleep, and so on.

Insomnia, difficulty falling asleep or staying asleep, affects about half of all cancer patients. As mentioned earlier, insomnia is frequently part of a cluster of symptoms that may include pain, fatigue, anxiety, and depression. Each of these medical problems, left untreated, has the potential to make the others worse: for example, poor sleep can contribute to a mood disturbance such as depression (think of women with postpartum depression who are sleep deprived), and someone who is depressed may have difficulty falling asleep or staying asleep because of sadness or worry. Furthermore, pain is one of the primary causes of insomnia, and appropriate treatment of pain can relieve not only the physical symptoms of pain and fatigue but also the emotional symptoms of depression and anxiety. In other cases, attempts to relieve pain can lead to or worsen symptoms of insomnia. (Some pain medications can cause daytime sleepiness, which may interfere with sleep at night, for instance.) Clearly a delicate balance is involved, and managing it requires the skill of an experienced physician.

There are many reasons that someone diagnosed with cancer might have insomnia. Since insomnia is common in the general population, it is not unusual for someone to have had difficulty with sleep before the cancer diagnosis. Insomnia is the most common sleep disorder, with up to 40 percent of the public reporting occasional difficulty and as much as 20 percent reporting persistent problems with sleep in the past year. But, even for those who have always slept well, the stress of a cancer illness may cause insomnia. Hospitalization, with its change in routine, its noise, its medication dosing schedules, and its unfamiliar environment, can encourage sleeplessness as well. Side effects from cancer therapy, too, including pain from surgery or other treatments, can make it difficult to fall asleep or stay asleep. Medications such as corticosteroids or therapy directed at decreasing hormone levels may impair one's ability to achieve a good night's rest. Circadian rhythms and the hormones and other chemical reactions related to the sleep-wake cycle may be affected by cancer and its therapies. For example, the concentrations of cytokines (such as tumor necrosis factor-alpha and interleukin-6), which play an important role in the sleep-wake cycle, can be altered in a person with cancer.

Regardless of whether a person has a history of insomnia, this problem can be caused or exacerbated by intense feelings of worry or sadness (anxiety or depression). Moreover, insomnia leads to daytime fatigue, which in turn can lead to napping during the day. Napping during the day often makes it more difficult to sleep at night—creating a vicious cycle of fatigue coupled with an inability to sleep well.

Although cancer-related fatigue is different from lethargy due to insomnia, inadequate sleep plays a role in the severity and continuation of cancer-related fatigue. Therefore, to improve energy levels, it is essential to identify sleep problems such as insomnia, sleep apnea (pauses in breathing during sleep), and periodic limb-movement disorder (also known as restless-leg syndrome).

Yet identifying sleep problems can be challenging since people are usually not able to give an accurate description of what happens to them at night. Nevertheless, sometimes what a patient says in the office is very revealing: "I am so tired, I think something is wrong with me." These words came from Susan, a young mother with two home-schooled daughters. Susan is busy all day teaching her girls and taking them out on field trips to museums, nature centers, and various other learning endeavors. By 8:00 p.m. her daughters are sound asleep and Susan gets energized. "After my kids are in bed is my best time of day. I don't feel tired at all." While the children sleep, she cleans her house, prepares meals for the next day, organizes the girls' lessons, watches TV, spends time with her husband, and uses the computer to catch up on emails. By 3:00 a.m., she is ready for bed. Susan's daughters are up by 8:00 a.m. and wake her with instant demands for help with dressing and breakfast requests.

This is a true story, though it might seem a little far-fetched. My point in sharing it is to highlight that sleep, or the lack thereof, and fatigue go hand in hand. It's simple: if you don't get enough sleep, you'll feel tired. You may be wondering how much sleep is enough. In an article titled "Sick and Tired: Does Sleep Have a Vital Role in the Immune System?," the authors note that the ideal amount of sleep for adults is approximately seven hours: "This duration is associated with the lower rate of morbidity [illness] and mortality. Both longer and shorter sleep durations are associated with increased risk." Keep in mind, though, that if you are actively undergoing cancer treatment, you may need more sleep than the average person.

If there is not a clear explanation for someone's fatigue or if a sleep problem is suspected, a sleep study is a good way to evaluate what is happening at night. Sleep studies, which can be done at home or in a hospital setting overnight, can provide a lot of objective information about how one sleeps. Among other things, a sleep study can determine how often a person moves (restless legs), whether there is a pause in breathing (apnea), whether the blood oxygen level dips during this pause, and whether the person moves through the stages of sleep appropriately. Although a sleep study is helpful in many instances, Table 9.4 lists specific signs that suggest a sleep study might be appropriate.

The next step in addressing a sleep problem is for a doctor to determine whether medication side effects or other medical issues (hot flashes, pain, anxiety, etc.) are contributing to the problem. Treatment will be based on the specific diagnosis and contributing factors, and it may involve adding or subtracting medications or prescribing devices to overcome causes of sleep disturbance (for example, a mouth guard or a breathing machine such as a continuous positive airway pressure machine). Treatment also should emphasize "sleep hygiene," the steps people can take on their own at home to prepare for a good night's rest. The "rules" of sleep hygiene are listed in Table 9.5.

CHEMO BRAIN AND FATIGUE

Although "chemo brain" is technically called *mild cognitive impairment* (MCI) and is different from fatigue, there is no doubt that being tired can affect your ability to recall things and concentrate on the task at hand. Cancer survivors often think they have MCI when in fact they are probably just exhausted. This is actually very important, because

Table 9.4. Reasons to Suspect the Presence of Sleep Apnea

During the Night
  Snoring
  Breathing pauses witnessed by bed partner
  Choking or gasping
  Restless sleep
  Dry mouth
  Drooling
  Awakening to urinate
  Heartburn (gastroesophogeal reflux)

During the Day
  Excessive daytime sleepiness
  Aggressiveness, irritability, depression, anxiety
  Decreased libido (sexual interest)
  Impotence
  Impaired memory or concentration
  Morning headache
  Morning sore throat

Physical Findings
  Obesity
  Deviated nasal septum (often associated with having had a broken nose)
  Large neck circumference
  Large tongue
  Narrow chin
  Abnormal mouth opening or closing

their cognitive abilities are intact. For an accurate diagnosis of MCI, there must be cognitive deficits that affect attention, memory, and concentration that are not a result of fatigue. However, the symptoms of MCI may be subtle, and cancer survivors often say that they feel fatigued, confused, mentally "foggy," or forgetful or they have difficulty concentrating and remembering. Importantly, both fatigue and MCI may be caused by some of the same medical problems, including anemia, cardiac or respiratory dysfunction, stress, depression, sleep disorders, and so on. MCI may occur in anyone who is undergoing or has

Table 9.5. The Rules of Good Sleep Hygiene

Manage Your Bedtime Routine

Go to bed only when you are tired.

Use your bedroom for sleep and sex only (not to watch television, etc.).

Arrange your bedroom environment so that it is quiet and dark and the temperature is moderate.

Try to establish regular times for going to bed and waking up.

Plan to get 7–8 hours of sleep at night.

Get rid of your bedroom clock (or hide it if you need the alarm for the morning).

Get out of bed and go to another room after 20–30 minutes (estimate this) if you are unable to sleep.

Avoid Things That Interfere with Sleep

Don't eat a heavy meal near bedtime.

Avoid drinking a lot of fluids.

Stop drinking caffeine at least 4–6 hours before bedtime.

Eliminate nicotine before bedtime.

Avoid alcohol after dinner (4–6 hours before bedtime).

Try not to exercise within 2 hours of bedtime (some say 6 hours).

Don't watch television or play computer games before bed.

Avoid naps during the day.

Be aware that sleeping pills are often effective only when used for a short period of time (2–4 weeks) and that some sleeping pills can actually make a sleep problem worse.

Relax before Bed

Taking a hot bath (not a shower) may promote sleep.

A light bedtime snack such as a glass of warm milk or a bowl of cereal can help.

Allow at least an hour before bedtime to unwind—read a book or listen to music.

Practice relaxation techniques such as biofeedback, meditation, deep breathing, imagery, etc.

had chemotherapy. Bed rest does not seem to improve the symptoms of MCI, and if there a history of sleep problems, these problems should be corrected prior to diagnosing MCI to determine whether the cognitive problems improve with proper rest.

EVALUATION OF FATIGUE

Because physicians often underestimate the amount of fatigue patients are experiencing and the impact it has on their ability to function (with cancer, the focus is on life-saving measures first and foremost), patients who are troubled by fatigue need to broach the subject with their doctors and inform them how fatigue is affecting their quality of life and ability to heal. Basically, if you don't tell your doctor, she or he won't know. Without your report there is no way to assess fatigue—it is a subjective symptom for which there is no accurate way to test in a typical office visit. Therefore, the first step in the evaluation of fatigue is for patients to describe what they are experiencing. A physical examination might give some clues as to the cause. For example, an anemic patient may have an increased heart rate (the heart has to pump faster to deliver more blood if there are fewer red blood cells to carry oxygen to the tissues) and a decreased capillary refill (when a finger is squeezed, it may take longer for the color to return). After taking a history of the symptoms and performing a physical examination, the doctor will decide whether to order tests and if so, which ones make the most sense. Table 9.6 provides a list of tests that may be included in a fatigue workup. The workup may be done in stages; the doctor might initially order some tests and based on those results determine what to do next (for example, order more tests or prescribe a specific treatment).

TREATMENT OF FATIGUE

In 1796 Thomas Ball submitted a dissertation to the Philadelphia Medical Society on "the causes and effects of sleep." Ball (who was about to become a doctor) suggested a number of remedies to "produce sedative effects." First on his list was bloodletting (a formerly popular procedure in which a small incision is made in a vein and some blood is removed from the sick person), which he stated "should be preferred to all other depleting remedies; because we have it more under command than any other." He elaborated by saying, "I have seen it necessary to bleed as oft as four, five, or even six times, before the excitement would be sufficiently reduced to admit of sleep." Other remedies he discussed included purging, vomiting, taking a cold bath, and inducing blisters.

Table 9.6. Screening Tests That May Be Done in a Fatigue Workup

Laboratory blood tests
    Complete blood count
    Erythrocyte sedimentation rate test
    Creatinine and urea nitrogen test
    Glucose test
    Calcium and phosphorus test
    Electrolyte test
    Albumin and total protein test
    Liver function tests
    Thyroid function tests
    Rheumatology screen
    C-reactive protein test
    Viral titers (Lyme, HIV, Epstein-Barr, etc.)
Urinalysis
Chest x-ray
Echocardiogram or electrocardiogram
Sleep study

Although Dr. Ball's remedies are well left in the past, we can commend him for recognizing the importance of sleep in health and disease.

Today the medical and pharmacological treatment of fatigue depends on the underlying reasons for the symptom. For instance, insomnia (caused by pain) and anemia are two common problems that cancer survivors face that contribute to fatigue. These problems, once identified, are usually easily resolved. For example, some cancer treatments cause hormonal fluctuations that may lead to insomnia: women with breast or endometrial cancer and men with prostate cancer may be affected by hot flashes, which can keep them awake at night. The cancer treatment may need to be continued, despite this bothersome side effect. A recent review published in the *Journal of the American Medical Association* reported that cognitive behavioral therapies often work as well as medications when it comes to treating insomnia. There are different types of cognitive behavioral therapies that may help with insomnia, including but not limited to sleep hygiene education (refer to Table 9.5), stimulus control and sleep restriction therapy (this involves strategies such as avoiding naps and keeping a regular sleep schedule), relaxation training (for example, guided imagery or progressive muscle relaxation), and cognitive therapy (such as avoiding unhelpful fears and ruminating about negative thoughts).

There are many prescription medications that may help with the fatigue. Describing the pharmacological treatment of fatigue for the problems that may cause one to not sleep well is beyond the scope of this chapter, but it is an important topic to discuss with your doctor. Some medications treat the sleep disorder while others may treat symptoms such as hot flashes, pain, or depression. Occasionally psychostimulants such as Ritalin are used during the day to help people have better alertness, attention, and focus. Here is a stepwise plan for addressing the symptom of fatigue:

Step 1. Make an appointment with your doctor to discuss your symptoms. Be sure to talk about how fatigue is affecting you on a daily basis. Describe any pain that you have and what your mood is like. Talk about your sleep pattern. Mention how often you exercise, what you are doing for exercise, and the intensity and duration of your fitness program. Describe your diet—how often you eat and what you eat. Tell your doctor about your use of alcoholic beverages. Make a list of all of your medications and any over-the-counter supplements you are taking, so that he or she can easily review it. Your doctor may order tests to further investigate your symptoms or suggest that you change your exercise regimen, bedtime routine, diet, and so forth. Schedule a follow-up appointment for one to two months later. At that time repeat this same process and note any changes you have made to improve your symptoms. Report how these changes have helped (or not). Specifically ask for further advice about treating your fatigue. Continue this pattern every couple of months until your symptoms improve and you are feeling more energetic.

Step 2. Exercise most days of the week; focus on aerobic (cardiovascular) exercise to improve your endurance and overall fitness level. Exercise has been shown to relieve fatigue in people with different kinds of cancer and is an easy way to both increase your energy and help your body to heal in other ways. While this may not seem intuitive, resting too much has been shown to contribute to cancer-related fatigue rather than lessen it. Therefore, if you are tired, try increasing your activity level instead of resting more.

Step 3. Exercise is important, but so is pacing yourself. Keep in mind that running errands and doing "busy work" is not helpful when it comes to physical healing. Therefore, as you focus on pursuing an appropriate exercise program, avoid overdoing it with chores that are energy depleting. Chapter 4 covers this topic in much greater detail.

Step 4. Eat a healthy diet and include frequent snacks as energy boosters. Maintaining your blood sugar level throughout the day is important. See chapter 8 for tips on how to eat to heal.

Step 5. Reduce your stress, anxiety, and depression. If you are feeling worried or sad, you can do things on your own or with the help of your doctor or mental health professional to improve your mood. Cognitive behavioral therapies may help a lot with this. Read chapter 11 for more about mood management.

Step 6. Sleep well. This may seem obvious, but it is important to remember: you will never feel energetic if you don't sleep well. Sleep is the way your body refreshes itself. If you don't sleep well in terms of quality *and* quantity, you'll feel tired. It's as simple as that. If you aren't sleeping well, talk to your doctor, who can help identify the problem and find possible solutions.

One way to evaluate your sleep is to keep a log for a week. What time do you go to bed and when do you wake up? Do you sleep all night? If not, what interferes with your sleep? Is your sleep restless? Do you feel refreshed in the morning? Also record how active you are during the day and whether you stop to rest or nap. The log will help you to determine whether what you do during the day affects your ability to sleep at night.

Fatigue can range from extremely debilitating to simply annoying. It is a frequent complaint in the general population—most people would like to have more energy. A cancer survivor's fatigue may be worse than what is experienced by others, and it can impair physical recovery because energy is a critical component in healing well. This is why proper rest is the third essential healing component in my list in chapter 2. Taking the time to evaluate and treat the troubling symptom of fatigue is worthwhile. The more energy you have, the better you will be able to tolerate cancer treatment and to heal.

References

C. S. Denlinger, J. A. Ligibel, M. Are, K. S. Baker, W. Demark-Wahnefried, D. L. Friedman, M. Goldman, L. Jones, A. King, G. H. Ku, et al. "Survivorship: Fatigue, Version 1. *Journal of the National Comprehensive Cancer Network* 12, no. 6 (June 2014): 876–87.

"Patient and Caregiver Resources," National Comprehensive Cancer Network, http://www.nccn.org/patients/resources/life_with_cancer/managing _symptoms/fatigue.aspx, accessed November 3, 2014.

X. S. Wang, F. Zhao, M. J. Fisch, A. M. O'Mara, D. Cella, T. R. Mendoza, and C. S. Cleeland, "Prevalence and Characteristics of Moderate to Severe Fatigue: A Multicenter Study in Cancer Patients and Survivors," *Cancer* 120, no. 3 (February 1, 2014): 425–32.

R. J. Reiter, "Melatonin: Clinical Relevance," *Best Practice and Research Clinical Endocrinology and Metabolism* 17 (2003): 273–85.

Mariangela Rondanelli, Milena Anna Faliva, Simone Perna, and Neldo Antoniello. "Update on the Role of Melatonin in the Prevention of Cancer Tumorigenesis and in the Management of Cancer Correlates, Such as Sleep-Wake and Mood Disturbances: Review and Remarks," *Aging Clinical and Experimental Research* 25, no. 5 (2013): 499–510.

S. Ancoli-Israel, "Sleep Is Not Tangible or What the Hebrew Tradition Has to Say about Sleep," *Psychosomatic Medicine* 63 (2001): 778–87.

P. A. Bryant et al., "Sick and Tired: Does Sleep Have a Vital Role in the Immune System?" *Nature Reviews Immunology* 4 (June 2004): 457–67.

T. Ball, "An Inaugural Dissertation on the Causes and Effects of Sleep" (MD diss., University of Pennsylvania, 1796), p. 2.

D. J. Buysse. "Insomnia" *Journal of the American Medical Association* 309, no. 7 (February 20, 2013): 706–16.

{ CHAPTER 10

EASE

YOUR PAIN }

There are a few illnesses that don't involve pain. Cancer isn't one of them. Pain is a part of cancer from the disease itself to its treatments. Treating pain in cancer patients is a priority. Recently, pain has become a major focus in treating *most* medical conditions—so much so that in a typical office medical practice, approximately eight of every ten visits are for conditions in which pain is present. In the hospital setting there are new guidelines for treating pain. I wrote about this topic in my book *Chronic Pain and the Family*:

> It's no secret that treating patients' pain adequately has not always been a priority in the hospital setting. The medical community is beginning to recognize the importance of treating acute pain, so much so that pain is now considered the "fifth" vital sign, after temperature, pulse, respiratory rate, and blood pressure. When hospitals undergo accreditation, they must show documentation that during admission patients' vital signs are taken and they are asked whether they are in pain. According to the *Comprehensive Accreditation Manual for Hospitals: The Official Handbook*, "The following statement on pain management is posted in all patient care areas (patient rooms, clinic rooms, waiting rooms, etc.). . . . All patients have a right to pain relief."

For many years, it was generally accepted that people with cancer would have to endure terrible pain. Unfortunately, this belief reflected the reality of the time, and cancer became almost synonymous with excruciating pain. Treatments for both pain and cancer have improved, however, and healthcare providers have become more cognizant of the importance of controlling pain not only to alleviate unnecessary suffering but also to promote healing. The notion that cancer patients are destined to suffer has now been relegated to the past.

Such progress doesn't mean that pain no longer exists. It certainly does, and we don't always have ways to control it adequately without problematic side effects. Although most doctors spend much of their time treating pain, few have had extensive training in this field of medicine. Oncologists typically are trained to treat pain related to the cancer itself but frequently have not had a lot of training in relieving musculoskeletal types of pain that may result from, say, scar tissue from surgery. Doctors in my specialty are often called "pain doctors" because they have extensive training in pain medicine, particularly for musculoskeletal problems. However, physiatrists usually don't have wide experience treating pain that is directly related to the location and spread of cancer.

Malignant Pain

Joe is a spry man in his 80s who still skis, sails, and works out at the gym. In his early 70s he was diagnosed with incurable prostate cancer. Despite the lack of a cure, many men diagnosed with prostate cancer live a long time with relatively few complications from this illness. When Joe was diagnosed, his doctors told him he would likely live a long and active life, and he is carrying out their prediction. Like many others with prostate cancer, Joe has to deal with some side effects of the hormonal treatment that slows the advancement of the disease. Loss of facial hair, voice changes, and decreased libido and sexual performance are among his side effects. Although they are unpleasant, Joe says that his main concern is controlling the pain from the cancer itself. For Joe, as for most people who have pain from incurable cancer, it is reasonable to treat him with daily opioid medications. These prescription drugs are usually given to cancer patients fairly liberally.

Opioids have a bad reputation among some people because this class of medications is notorious for abuse. I explored this issue in detail in the book I wrote on pain:

Opium is a naturally occurring substance that comes from poppy juice. It contains a number of chemicals such as morphine and codeine. Some opioids are also synthetically made in the laboratory. These potent pain-killers, whether they occur naturally or are synthetically produced, attach to specific proteins called opioid receptors (which are found in the brain, spinal cord, and gastrointestinal tract) and block the transmission of pain messages to the brain.

Opioids can be taken safely and are the mainstay of pain treatment for cancer that is not curable. It is essential that I convey to readers the following message: *addiction problems with opioids are usually only a concern in patients who do not currently have cancer*. If you have pain from the cancer, opioids are a very reasonable class of medications to take.

The World Health Organization suggests a stepwise "ladder" approach to the use of pain medications. Step 1 on the ladder involves giving nonopioid medications such as anti-inflammatory drugs. In step 2 an opioid (such as codeine, dihydrocodeine, or tramadol) is added for mild to moderate pain. Step 3 is for when the patient has moderate to severe pain and doesn't receive enough relief from step 2. In step 3 the physician prescribes a "stronger" opioid (for example, morphine) instead of the "weaker" opioids used in step 2.

Studies have shown that sometimes there is a mismatch of expectations between patients and their doctors and nurses when it comes to opioid prescriptions. Patients may believe they can safely take high doses of these drugs, while the doctors and other healthcare professionals who are administering them might be concerned about the risk of serious side effects at higher doses. Tables 10.1 and 10.2 list the potential problems associated with opioid medications. If you have considerable pain from cancer, don't let these lists frighten you. As I mentioned, oncologists tend to be very knowledgeable about this class of drugs; your doctor should be able to help you to achieve significant (though not necessarily complete) pain relief while avoiding complications from opioids.

Sometimes opioids are used in cancer treatment in conjunction with other medications. For example, if someone has a tumor that is pressing on a nerve, then a medication such as gabapentin, which is in the class of antiseizure drugs but is often used for nerve pain, might be a

Table 10.1. Potential Problems with Opioid Medications

Side Effects

Serious side effects of opioids can include respiratory depression (slowed breathing), so it's recommended that these medications not be used in conjunction with alcohol, antihistamines, barbiturates, or benzodiazepines. (There are exceptions; if you are taking opioids, just be sure to tell your doctor about any other medications you're taking that can be sedating or cause respiratory depression.) Other side effects may include rash or itching, nausea with or without vomiting, constipation, sedation, dizziness, cognitive impairment, and difficulty urinating.

Tolerance

Tolerance occurs when someone requires an increased dose of medication to experience the same level of pain relief (that is, after many doses, the drug becomes less effective in managing pain).

Physical Dependence

Physical dependence results in symptoms of withdrawal when the medication is abruptly discontinued. It occurs after more than just a few days of continuous use. Physical dependence is usually not a problem as long as patients are told to wean themselves off these medications rather than stopping abruptly. Drug dependence and tolerance are both physical problems. They *do not* indicate either addiction or abuse.

Addiction

Addiction is characterized by a compulsive use and craving of any substance that is used for mood-altering purposes. Individuals are addicted to opioids (or any other drug) if they (1) lose control over the use of the medication, (2) use the medication compulsively, (3) crave the medication, and (4) continue to take the medication despite the possibility of harm to themselves or others. In other words, addiction is a medical condition that manifests itself as a psychological and behavioral problem.

Abuse

Abuse means using a substance in a way that deviates from approved medical use or social patterns within society. Abuse is subject to cultural disapproval and is often associated with the "recreational" use of substances. Approximately one-third of the U.S. population has used illicit drugs. It is estimated that 6%–15% of the population has some form of substance-use disorder. People are most familiar with abuse in the context of illegal street drugs; however, estimates indicate that up to 28% of controlled substances are abused. Moreover, according to estimates, more than 4 million Americans use prescription drugs for nonmedical purposes. Prescription medications are often "diverted" from legitimate channels to illicit ones via falsified prescriptions.

Table 10.2. Signs of Opioid Withdrawal Compared to Signs of Intoxication

Withdrawal	
Increase in saliva and tears	Muscle cramps
Yawning	Drug craving
Enlarged pupils	Bad mood
Gooseflesh	*Intoxication*
Tremors	Insensitivity to pain
Inability to sleep	Drowsiness
Decreased appetite	Euphoria
Vomiting	Mental clouding
Diarrhea	Constricted pupils
Irritability	Vomiting
Increased blood pressure	Difficulty breathing

reasonable option. Other times opioids are used with antidepressant medications that affect serotonin levels or other substances (that help modulate pain) in the brain.

Although opioids are a mainstay in the treatment of pain from a malignancy, there are many other possible medications—some of which not only can alleviate pain but also may slow the growth of the cancer. For example, in many types of advanced cancer, the disease spreads (metastasizes) to the bones. The class of bisphosphonate medications may be helpful in treating the associated pain as well as reducing the risk of fracture, though the current research is far from conclusive and these drugs are not typically given to cancer patients for pain. This class of medications has been used in research studies looking at breast, prostate, and lung cancer as well as myeloma (bone marrow cancer) and other cancers. In a recent review on the use of bisphosphonates in men with advanced prostate cancer, the researchers noted that skeletal complications due to bone loss may be associated with not only severe pain but also decreased survival (this may be due to falls involving fractures and medically associated complications), reduced quality of life, and increased healthcare costs. Bisphosphonates and other medications (such as denosumab) may help prevent bone loss and reduce pain as well as other complications.

There are many other ways to treat cancer pain, thereby enhancing the person's quality and possibly length of life. For example, external beam radiation and surgery are treatments that can shrink tumors. Radiopharmaceuticals, though not commonly used for bone pain, are drugs that can be administered intravenously and may be an option for someone with cancer in the bones. Corticosteroid injections in the spinal region or other areas can help to alleviate pain. The list of options is extensive and continually expanding. Appropriate treatment depends on the type and stage of cancer as well as the areas affected and the associated pain symptoms. Patient and physician preference for a particular treatment choice is also an important consideration.

The use of cannabinoids (such as marijuana) in the treatment of cancer has received quite a bit of press. Cannabinoids have been shown to be helpful treatments in cancer and can improve appetite, reduce nausea and vomiting, and alleviate pain. When cannabis is used medically, it may take various forms; often it is dissolved in sesame oil and then swallowed in gelatin capsules. Cannabinoid smoke may be a risk factor for respiratory cancers, so this form is not used.

NONMALIGNANT PAIN

Practically everyone who has ever had cancer has an almost unconscious pain filter that works something like this: "Hey, I have a pain in my [fill in the body part]. Could this be a recurrence?" What they really want to know is whether this is a "safe" pain or something that could be life threatening.

Chloe is a middle-aged woman who had endometrial cancer more than a decade ago. At the time, she had a number of pelvic lymph nodes removed and subsequently developed problems with lymph drainage that resulted in swelling of her right leg (called lymphedema). This swelling was painless, and for many years Chloe wasn't overly concerned about recurrence of her cancer. However, over time she began to experience increasing back pain. Chloe immediately thought that her cancer had come back and spread to her spine. During her initial office visit, it was clear to me that her back pain was likely due to the awkward position in which she slept, with her leg elevated to minimize the swelling. Of course, I ordered the appropriate imaging tests just to be sure there was no cancer, and they came back normal. I recommended that

Chloe meet with one of our therapists who is certified in the treatment of lymphedema for better management that didn't involve awkward sleep positions. In a few weeks, Chloe's back pain went away.

Nonmalignant pain is common in cancer survivors for a number of reasons. People often have postoperative pain problems related to a surgery and resultant scar tissue. It is not uncommon to have postoperative complications such as arm or leg swelling due to lymphedema (which is usually painless but can cause pain, for example, if the swelling is severe and compresses a nerve or if people overuse their "good" arm or leg and develop pain in this limb). Injury to the brain or spinal cord can cause weakness and structural problems with resultant pain. Lack of activity while a person is ill and during convalescence can lead to reduced strength, which might promote such problems as back and neck pain.

FINE-TUNING YOUR PAIN FILTER

As I mentioned, nearly all cancer survivors have what I call a very sensitive pain filter. What a person might have ignored in the past now becomes a concern: Is that cancer pain I am feeling? Fine-tuning your pain filter and recognizing when to seek medical advice can contribute to your peace of mind. Since most new pain will go away within two weeks, I usually advise people to monitor their discomfort over this period and, if it persists, to seek help then. Here's some advice on adjusting your pain filter:

1. Pain that is new, unidentified, or severe and occurs in the chest, abdomen, or head should be investigated as soon as possible. This is not necessarily a cancer issue, but it could indicate a heart attack or some other serious problem.
2. Pain that is accompanied by other symptoms such as numbness, weakness, and dizziness should be investigated as soon as possible. Again, this is not necessarily a cancer issue, but it may indicate some other serious problem.
3. Pain that is caused by trauma (for example, pain after a car accident or a fall from a ladder) should be attended to immediately, regardless of whether there is acute bleeding.

4. Most pain that people experience is musculoskeletal in origin. Musculoskeletal pain, such as that affecting the extremities, the neck, and the low back (muscular strains, tendinitis, arthritis, etc.), is usually not terribly serious. This is why it is usually reasonable to wait two weeks to see if the pain disappears. Even if the pain doesn't go away, there is a very good chance that it is not cancer related. So, persistent pain should not necessarily alarm you but rather prompt you to seek out an appropriate diagnosis and treatment.

5. As you fine-tune your pain filter, remember that cancer pain is not typically intermittent. It doesn't usually come and go and wax and wane to a great degree. Rather, tumors that grow to the point of being painful are pressing on structures that elicit pain. They often cause night pain and awaken people from their sleep. The pain doesn't tend to change or go away for a while. Instead, cancer pain is the kind of persistent pain that makes you take notice.

6. A doctor who can assess the problem and order appropriate tests should evaluate any pain that you experience.

7. Finally, bear in mind that being pain-free is usually a temporary condition. Most of us live with minor aches and pains, which occur for a variety of reasons. To prove this, you could take a poll of your colleagues or friends. Ask them whether they have experienced any one of these three conditions in the past few weeks: (1) low back pain, (2) neck pain, or (3) headache. Most adults will say yes. So, although your pain filter may be working overtime, do keep in mind that most pain conditions are relatively benign.

PHARMACOLOGICAL OPTIONS FOR NONMALIGNANT PAIN

Nonmalignant pain may be classified as *nociceptive* or *neuropathic*. Nociceptive pain occurs when the tissues have been injured and an immune response causes swelling and other injury-healing actions. With neuropathic pain, there may be direct or indirect trauma to nerves. For example, some chemotherapeutic agents are toxic to nerves in the hands and feet and can cause a peripheral neuropathy that may be quite painful. Pharmacological options usually come in one of three forms: topical medications such as creams or patches, oral medications (pills or liquid preparations), and injections. Most doctors have experience treating pain with oral medications and sometimes topical drugs, and a pain specialist is usually knowledgeable about prescribing oral and topical drugs and skilled at performing injections.

Nociceptive pain is usually treated with oral anti-inflammatory medications and with analgesics (drugs that alleviate pain, such as acetaminophen or in some cases opioids). If there is associated muscle spasm, muscle relaxants may be helpful. The use of opioids for nonmalignant pain, particularly if it is relatively protracted and not due to an acute injury, is controversial and beyond the scope of this text. Neuropathic pain generally responds better to medications that influence chemicals involved in nerve signal transmission. The most common classes of medications that help to alleviate neuropathic pain are antidepressant and antiseizure drugs. Table 10.3 lists the types of oral medications commonly prescribed for nonmalignant pain and some of their potential side effects.

Medications can also be given topically or injected. Topical pain medications include lidocaine patches, which contain a local anesthetic that can numb a painful area. Capsaicin is a commercially available pepper-based cream that can provide pain relief. Some creams are commercially available with a prescription while others require a

Table 10.3. Medications Commonly Used for Nonmalignant Pain and Their Potential Side Effects	
Acetaminophen	Liver damage
Tramadol hydrochloride	Nausea, vomiting, dry mouth, dizziness, sedation
NSAIDs (nonsteroidal anti-inflammatory drugs)*	Gastrointestinal bleeding, injury to the kidneys, increased blood pressure
Muscle relaxants	Dizziness, sedation, constipation, blood or liver injury
Lidocaine 5% patch	Skin irritation or rash
Antidepressants	Sedation, dry mouth, constipation, inability to urinate, weight gain
Antiseizure drugs	Dizziness, nausea, blood or liver injury, sedation, weight gain

compounding pharmacist to make creams that contain combinations of these medications—depending on the patient's needs. Pharmacists who are skilled in making compounds can take almost any oral medication and turn it into a cream, thereby usually lessening the side effects. Topical drugs often don't have the same absorption as oral medications, so their therapeutic effect may be reduced as well. Examples of drugs that can be made into creams include anti-inflammatory medications, antidepressants, antiseizure drugs, muscle relaxants, and opioids.

Pain medicine can be injected around or into painful areas (see Table 10.4). There are many different kinds of injections; some of the more common ones include injections into muscle trigger points, joints, and areas of the spine, and injections around tendons. Nerve blocks are injections that can be administered essentially anywhere that a nerve is causing pain. Botulinum toxin, cosmetically used for wrinkles, also has some medical pain applications. This drug has surprisingly few side effects and is one of the safest methods of treating pain if administered by an expert. There is anecdotal evidence that botulinum toxin injections may alleviate postmastectomy pain. There are many other pain uses of this drug as well.

NONPHARMACOLOGICAL TREATMENT OPTIONS: EXERCISE

There are also many nonpharmacological ways to treat pain (see Table 10.5). Exercise is one of the most important methods. Many instances of pain begin with a muscular imbalance, poor posture, and poor alignment of the skeletal structure. For example, people with low back pain often have poor posture, weak abdominal muscles, and tight hamstring muscles. Many musculoskeletal problems can arise during or after cancer treatment. Pain causes people to become increasingly sedentary; inactivity leads to a poorer physical condition, which in turn leads to yet more pain. Exercise also offers enormous psychological benefits that can enhance a person's ability to function.

When treating pain, doctors often send patients to physical therapy, occupational therapy, or both to learn specific exercises. Because many conditions can worsen with the wrong type of exercise, I typically refer patients to expert therapists who can show them what to do for their particular problem. A good therapist appreciates the differ-

Table 10.4. Common Types of Injections to Treat Nonmalignant Pain	
Trigger-point injections	Medication is administered in specific areas of the muscle that are pain generators (for fibromyalgia, muscle pain syndromes, etc.).
Tendon injections	Medication is injected around, but not into, the tendon (for tendinitis, lateral epicondylitis, etc.).
Nerve blocks	Medication is injected near, but not into, the nerve (for reflex sympathetic dystrophy, carpal tunnel syndrome, spinal nerve compression syndromes, etc.).
Epidural injections	Medication is delivered to the epidural space in the spine (for spinal stenosis and lumbar or cervical radiculopathy from a herniated disk).
Facet blocks	Injections are performed around the facet joints in the spine for relief of pain usually due to arthritis of the facet joint itself (for cervical facet and lumbar facet arthritis).
Botulinum toxin injections	Botulinum toxin is injected directly into the muscles to decrease muscle spasm or spasticity (for spinal cord injury, stroke, migraine headaches, etc.).
Joint injections	Medication is injected into the joint space (for knee arthritis, sacroiliac joint pain, etc.).
Bursitis injections	If the bursa is inflamed, the first part of the procedure may involve draining the fluid and the second part injecting medication to reduce inflammation (for shoulder bursitis, hip bursitis, etc.).

Table 10.5. Nonpharmacological Treatment Options for Nonmalignant Pain	
Assistive devices (for example, canes)	Massage
Biofeedback	Meditation
Braces	Modalities such as hot and cold packs
Ergonomic equipment (for example, a telephone ear set)	Relaxation therapy
Exercise	Stress reduction
Footwear or orthotics	Transcutaneous electrical nerve stimulation (TENS)
Guided imagery	
Hypnosis	Ultrasound

ent types of exercises (flexibility, strengthening, and cardiovascular or aerobic exercises) and chooses specific exercises from each category that will promote reconditioning and healing. These targeted exercises that are designed to treat the pain from *physical impairments* are called *therapeutic exercise* and should be prescribed by healthcare professionals such as physical or occupational therapists. Like all practitioners, therapists vary in their skill levels and interests, so it is essential to work with someone who is skilled at treating people with your particular condition. If people are very sedentary, I usually encourage them to begin exercising on their own at the same time—even if it just means a 5-minute walk (see chapter 7).

Massage

The use of massage to treat a cancer survivors is controversial. In the past, there was concern that massage may increase the blood supply to a particular area, which might support tumor growth. But there is also the theory that massage may be helpful. In a study published in the *International Journal of Neuroscience*, researchers found that women diagnosed with breast cancer who received massage therapy reported less depression, anxiety, and pain. These women also had an increase in dopamine, natural killer cells, and lymphocytes, which may indicate an increased immune response—theoretically somewhat helpful in treating cancer or preventing recurrence. Use of therapeutic ultrasound, a form of deep heat, has been the subject of similar concerns. But some scientists think ultrasound actually diminishes tumor growth. I recommend that you talk to your doctor about these two therapies, if you are considering using them. Until we know more, I generally recommend avoiding massage or ultrasound over a site where there is currently a tumor, and I hesitate to recommend their use directly over a site where a tumor was located in the past.

Other Modalities

Modalities are treatments that can be applied to a painful area of the body. Hot and cold packs are modalities that can be used at home. Caution is needed, though, because both heat and cold can cause serious tissue damage if applied for too long or if the temperature is extreme.

Hot and cold packs should usually not be directly applied to the skin. Cold packs should not be left on for more than 20 minutes at a time, and there should be a break of at least an hour between treatments. Cold packs also should not be applied to the extremities of people who have problems with circulation (for example, peripheral vascular disease). Ice massage can also be an effective method of relieving pain. You can freeze a paper cup filled with water and then cut the cup to expose the ice. Then apply it to the affected area with a circular motion. Because you are moving the ice around and not leaving it stationary on the skin, you can have direct contact of the ice and skin.

Another home-based remedy is transcutaneous electrical nerve stimulation (TENS), which is administered by a unit with electrodes that stick to the skin. This device is often first used in physical therapy to assess whether it is helpful in relieving the pain. TENS units are compact (similar in size to a cell phone) and can be easily hidden under one's clothes. They are typically worn intermittently during the day. Interferential units are similar to TENS. Occasionally this is used for chronic pain, but it tends to work better for acute pain issues such as the reduction of swelling. Neither unit is recommended for use directly over a tumor because of the potential risk of stimulating malignant cells.

Other modalities are more sophisticated, and therapists receive special training to use them. Among them are electrical stimulation, ultrasound (a deep-heating technique that is usually not recommended for people with cancer), and iontophoresis. In iontophoresis electrical impulses are used to apply topical corticosteroids; the medication penetrates the skin, but the skin is not broken. This procedure is sometimes preferred over injections, which do break the skin. In people with dark skin, corticosteroids (whether applied on the surface of the skin or beneath the surface) can cause lightening of the skin in the region they are used. There are some precautions that need to be taken with various modalities (for example, ultrasound); the prescribing physician and the therapist should be aware of these.

Physical and occupational therapists often perform what is generally termed "manual therapy": joint and soft-tissue mobilization techniques to aid with pain reduction through normalizing the alignment of bones and the surrounding soft tissues. Decreasing muscle spasm using hands-on "myofascial release" techniques further helps to normalize soft tissue and can lead to pain relief. These include craniosacral therapy, deep tissue massage, and muscle trigger-point massage.

Special Equipment

A great deal of equipment is available to help with pain relief, depending on the particular condition in question. For example, a telephone headset or ear set is ideal for someone with neck pain. If you have hand pain and need to use the computer, voice-activated software can be extremely helpful. For people with back pain or foot pain, custom shoe orthotics or extra-deep and extra-wide orthopedic shoes can provide relief. And if you have hip or knee pain, a cane can reduce the load borne by the affected joint, diminishing the pain. There are so many types of equipment that it is impossible to discuss them all here. But the right equipment is incredibly important when treating pain.

A long-standing patient of mine, Sam, discovered this when he came to see me with severe ankle arthritis that made every step excruciating. Sam told me that he had been to see an orthopedic surgeon who had recommended an ankle fusion to relieve the pain. Sam had decided against the surgery, because he had heart disease and was worried he wouldn't make it through the operation. I told Sam that there was a good chance he could be fitted with a special brace (called an ankle foot orthosis) that would completely relieve his pain. Sam was doubtful that it would help, but when he came to our brace clinic and tried the brace out, he couldn't believe that all of his pain disappeared.

This example not only illustrates the importance of the right equipment in treating pain; it also shows how getting a second opinion from a doctor who specializes in treating pain but is in a different medical specialty may provide you with additional treatment options.

Lifestyle Changes

Sometimes after cancer you have to make lifestyle changes whether you want to or not. I have an acquaintance who works as a housecleaner. Recently, she was diagnosed with cervical cancer and underwent surgery that included removing her uterus (hysterectomy). For several months while she recovered from the operation and received other treatment, she was unable to manage the physical aspects of cleaning homes for a living. Of course, many of us who have gone through cancer and its treatment have had to take time off from work—for either a short time or a long time.

Lifestyle changes don't have to be an "all-or-none" type of thing, however. The young woman who is a housecleaner was able to go back to work and avoid heavy lifting (carrying the vacuum cleaner up and down stairs) by having her sister help her out. Another one of my patients helped to solve her arm pain problems (they were most acute when she drove more than an hour each way to and from work) by getting her boss to agree to let her work from home part of the time.

One of the stores I used to frequent where you could buy products in bulk began to use automated self-checkout lines. I would not only take the heavy bulk items I wanted from the store's shelves and place them in my cart, but then I would lift them out to scan them at the checkout and place them back in my cart. I would load them into my car, and then finally I would carry them into the house and store them. I found myself dreading going to this store, and eventually I stopped altogether. Since I had shopped there for years, it took me a while to figure out that it just wasn't worth the cost savings to do all of this physical work, especially when I was trying to heal from cancer.

There are many lifestyle changes that can help relieve your pain and assist you in your efforts to heal. To learn what some of these might be, pay attention to what I call "the voice of your body." What is it telling you with respect to pain? What are you doing that is causing more pain? This is a key question, because whatever you are doing that makes your pain worse, you should try to modify or stop altogether. This principle applies to everyone who is experiencing pain, not just cancer survivors. One day a man in his fifties came to see me about his hip pain. He said, "You see, doctor, I have pain when I cross my leg like this. My x-rays are normal, so I know I don't have arthritis. Can you help me?" When I asked how often he crossed his leg in that particular fashion, he told me that he never really does but that once he did and he noticed it was painful. My advice was simple, "Don't cross your leg that way." This may seem flippant, and I certainly don't mean to make light of anyone's pain, but as a pain doctor, I always tell people to first consider how they might modify their lifestyle to avoid or limit those activities that exacerbate the pain. Sometimes a lifestyle modification is the cure.

Psychological Intervention

Once when I had a patient who complained of severe hand pain but had no objective findings (his physical examination, x-rays, and lab tests were completely normal), I sent him for a consultation with a colleague who specializes in treating chronic pain. My colleague concurred with my workup—he agreed that there was no identifiable reason for this man's pain. Yet we both believed that this patient was suffering. My colleague suggested a psychiatric consultation to evaluate and treat his anxiety. As I explained the reason for the referral to my patient, I told him that we did not believe the pain was "all in his head" but that his overall anxiety was affecting his ability to cope with the pain. Indeed, once his anxiety was under control, despite continued hand pain, he felt much better.

In pain treatment programs, a clinical social worker, a psychologist, and a psychiatrist may be available to help both the patient and the family deal with the emotional aspects of the problem. Psychiatrists usually focus on prescribing medications to alleviate depression and anxiety. Clinical social workers and psychologists can provide counseling and may use techniques such as guided imagery, hypnosis, therapeutic touch, and the like to decrease stress and improve a person's ability to deal with pain.

Surgery

Surgery is an excellent method of treatment for some pain problems; however, because of the potential for serious side effects, it should never be done without exploring other options. Especially for people healing from cancer and cancer treatment (which may have already involved surgery), unnecessary operations should be avoided. There are times when surgery is very helpful for such individuals, though. One of my patients is a woman with a history of breast cancer who now has lymphedema in her arm. The swelling in her arm and the constant use of her arm at work on the computer, coupled with a long commute to work in which she has to hold her hands in a certain position, have caused severe carpal tunnel syndrome (compression of the medial nerve at the wrist). Normally, surgery for carpal tunnel syndrome has a low risk of complications, but in someone with lymphedema there is a higher risk of potential problems such as worsening arm swelling and infection. When I referred this patient for surgery (which was very successful), she was experiencing terrible pain, which was at its worst when she drove to work. As a single woman with no other source of income, she needed to be able to work, and she wasn't in a position (after a recent bout with cancer) to look for a job closer to home and one that wouldn't involve repetitive use of her hands. So, in this patient, surgery was a very reasonable option. While operations work well in some cases, all surgeries are associated with significant risks. Therefore, for pain conditions that are not life threatening, other solutions should be explored and considered first.

COMPLEMENTARY PAIN THERAPIES

Complementary therapies may help with pain, and many are focused on relieving this symptom. As noted in chapter 6, complementary therapies are a reasonable option if the risks are minimal and the cost is not prohibitive. Many of these treatments that have been shown to be helpful in cancer patients are offered at hospitals and centers that have oncology clinics. For example, acupuncture and massage are frequently available to people undergoing cancer treatment. Be aware that neither of these treatments should *cause* pain. If it does, either the person performing the treatment is not skilled enough, or the person receiving the treatment is hypersensitive and this form of therapy is not a good option for him or her. Mind-body therapies (for example meditation and hypnosis) are also often available in cancer centers. If you are considering taking dietary supplements or botanicals for any reason, including pain relief, talk to your doctor about possible side effects and drug interactions.

Pain is depleting and may impair your ability to physically recover from cancer and cancer treatment. The approaches for malignant versus nonmalignant (usually musculoskeletal) pain are quite different. For malignant pain, your oncologist should be guiding your treatment.

For nonmalignant pain that persists, consider asking for a referral to a pain specialist such as a doctor who is trained in physical medicine and rehabilitation. Keep in mind that "toughing it out" when it comes to dealing with pain is not a wise course—especially if you are trying to heal. Instead, seek out professional help to alleviate your pain and continue on your road to recovery.

REFERENCES

J. Silver, *Chronic Pain and the Family* (Cambridge, MA: Harvard University Press, 2004), pp. 10, 104.

"WHO's Cancer Pain Ladder for Adults," World Health Organization, http://www.who.int/cancer/palliative/painladder/en/, accessed November 3, 2014.

M. Iranikhah, S. Stricker, and M. K. Freeman, "Future of Bisphosphonates and Denosumab for Men with Advanced Prostate Cancer," *Cancer Management and Research* 6 (May 3, 2014): 217–24.

M. Hernandez-Reif et al., "Natural Killer Cells and Lymphocytes Increase in Women with Breast Cancer Following Massage Therapy," *International Journal of Neuroscience* 115 (2005): 495–510.

{ CHAPTER 11

Monitor
Your Mood

}

Hamilton Jordan, the youngest presidential chief of staff in American history (he served in the Carter administration), survived three kinds of cancer before the age of 50. He titled his provocative memoir *No Such Thing as a Bad Day*. After living through non-Hodgkin's lymphoma, melanoma, and prostate cancer, Jordan considers himself a lucky man. If you read his memoir, however, you'll find that in fact he had many bad days as he was struggling to cure his cancers and regain his health. Everyone who is diagnosed with cancer has bad days. Even in the earliest stages, and in the best-case scenarios, the word *cancer* carries with it an ominous threat against our very survival. To be worried, sad, frustrated, frightened, and angry is normal when you have been told you have cancer. But prolonged worry and angst may have an ill effect on your ability to heal both physically and psychologically. In this chapter I want to help you figure out how you can best manage the emotional roller coaster of a cancer diagnosis.

I remember a lot of bad days during and after my treatment. One in particular stands out—a day when I thought I must have been inserted into someone else's life. One of my colleagues had taken a day off from work to escort me to chemotherapy. It was a long day, and when we were ready to leave, I was feeling nauseous, weak, and shaky. As I hobbled to the parking lot, my colleague began frantically searching for her minivan. Where had she parked it? Finally, we saw a similar vehicle next to the kiosk where you pay the attendant. But this van had the back window smashed and there was serious body damage to the rear door. We couldn't see the full extent of the damage because a long piece of plastic had been applied with duct tape across the broken glass in back. We looked at each other and immediately knew that this was her car. Apparently, while I was undergoing chemo, one of the parking attendants had attempted to move her car and had backed into a pole. On the long ride home in rush-hour traffic, we laughed about how bad the situation was. I had cancer. She was trying to help me and now her car was wrecked. It happened to be one of the coldest nights of the year in Boston. The plastic and the duct tape were whipping around and admitting plenty of outside air, so our teeth were chattering. To top it off, the parking attendant in the kiosk had made us pay to leave the garage! Although I was laughing, I was also thinking in a very heartbroken way, "This can't be my life . . ."

But it was my life and there would be other bad days. Everyone has them, of course, but people who have cancer might encounter a lot of bad days. Feeling as though your mood is not at your usual baseline is normal as you go through this experience. The last thing I want to do is to make anyone feel guilty or worried about how they are feeling. Instead, I want to help you understand the effect that your mood has on your recovery. Intermittent bad days, or even several weeks' worth of bad days all strung in a row, will likely have no effect on your health. Experiencing problems with your mood for more than a few weeks, though, might impact your ability to heal well and move on with your life.

THE LINK BETWEEN EMOTIONAL AND PHYSICAL HEALTH

Your emotional health is intimately related to your physical well-being, though we don't understand all of the effects that one has on the other. In 2007, there was a very important report released by the Institute of Medicine titled "Cancer Care for the Whole Patient: Meeting Psychosocial Health Needs." This report generated a lot of interest in further evaluating distress in cancer survivors. Since then, many research studies have been published, and not surprisingly these have demonstrated a strong link between physical and psychological health in cancer survivors. For example, in several studies the leading cause of distress was physical disability or decreased ability to physically function. In a study evaluating the health-related quality of life in cancer survivors, the researchers found that approximately one in four individuals had decreased quality of life due to physical problems whereas only one in ten had decreased quality of life due to emotional problems. The Institute of Medicine report along with new research studies encouraged the adoption of "distress screening" in hospitals and cancer centers throughout the United States. However, because physical problems frequently are the root cause of cancer survivors' distress, I have written extensively about the need not only for distress screening but also for physical impairment screening—what I call *dual screening*. Refer to Figure 5.1 to recall why dual screening is much better than distress screening alone.

Dr. Jimmie Holland is chief of psychiatry at Memorial Sloan-Kettering Cancer Center. In her book *The Human Side of Cancer: Living with Hope, Coping with Uncertainty*, she discusses many of the cancer myths as they pertain to the effect of emotions on physical health, including the following three:

1. You wanted to have cancer.
2. The problems from your difficult childhood caused it.
3. Your negative attitude is making the tumor grow faster.

Dr. Holland tells readers that these myths are harmful: "There is no scientific basis for these beliefs, which place an unconscionable added burden on patients who already have enough to cope with." Moreover, "for most patients, cancer is the most difficult and frightening experience they have ever encountered. All this hype claiming that if you don't have a positive attitude and that if you get depressed you are making your tumor grow faster invalidates people's natural and understandable reactions to a threat to their lives." Dr. Holland calls this the "tyranny of positive thinking."

I absolutely agree with Dr. Holland that "blame the victim" philosophies, prevalent for centuries and still sometimes part of the cancer culture, are unquestionably detrimental. However, Dr. Holland acknowledges the fascinating and growing field of *psychoneuroimmunol-*

ogy, which is the scientific study of the relationships among the brain, the hormone (endocrine) system, and the immune system. Research in this area of medicine has helped us better understand the real physical responses our bodies have to stress. We know that response to stress is important in heart disease, and we are learning more about how it might affect aberrant cell growth such as in malignancies. As Dr. Holland cautions, however, "People today have many questions, based on what they've read and what their friends tell them about cancer and the mind. And people make a lot of mistakes and premature assumptions on the basis of incomplete research."

When I was first diagnosed with cancer, I believed that I had a terrible prognosis. Several times over the course of two years I had tests done to check out an irregularity I noticed on my left breast. The first three doctors I saw didn't detect anything on either my mammogram or on two different ultrasounds of my breast. I began to feel like a hypochondriac. Finally, two years later, a second mammogram and a third ultrasound, together with a biopsy of a now noticeable tumor, confirmed my suspicion of breast cancer. I was terrified that the delay in my diagnosis meant that I had a poor prognosis.

With breast cancer, as with many other cancers, the staging (determining whether the disease is caught early or in a more advanced stage) is done as a result of the tissue taken at surgery. While I was awaiting surgery and information about the progression of my illness, I talked to the wife of one of my colleagues, who had been diagnosed with breast cancer. She told me that after she was diagnosed she was convinced she was going to die. This feeling lasted for several years. But over time these thoughts abated, and now, more than a decade after her initial diagnosis, she believes that her cancer won't come back. A patient of mine, a man in his 50s, was diagnosed with a rare type of cancer (fewer than seven hundred cases have been reported in the United States) that usually has a poor prognosis. He was told by his doctors to be sure that his estate was in order. Because he was the primary breadwinner and had many unpaid bills, he declared bankruptcy so that his wife wouldn't be left in a terrible financial situation. Yet, despite the odds and his preparations to die, he lived.

As I found out after I had surgery, my prognosis was better than

I initially suspected. The reason I share these stories is to show that pessimism, though perhaps not ideal, is not directly linked with disease progression, recurrence, or survival. Just because you think your cancer may kill you doesn't mean it will. Dr. Holland's "tyranny of positive thinking" is a way of saying that you don't have to be optimistic to survive cancer.

YOUR BASELINE MOOD

My mother and father had a deep and abiding love for each other, and, when my father died, my mother was truly despondent. I remember one conversation I had with her a few months after his death, when she told me about a TV interview of Dr. Joyce Brothers that she had seen. Dr. Brothers talked about how most of us have an emotional baseline, whether it's generally happy or chronically depressed or somewhere in between. When we suffer a terrible blow, for whatever reason, our emotional status can change. A generally optimistic person might become deeply pessimistic. A content person may feel discontented. A usually calm person may experience intense anxiety.

After a while, though (usually weeks to months but sometimes years), most people return to their previous emotional baseline. My mother has had this experience. Though she still grieves over losing my father, emotionally she is back where she feels most comfortable, rather calm and typically optimistic.

A cancer diagnosis is not only a threat to your life but also a threat to your well-being. Though there are many factors we don't understand about how one's mood may affect *quantity* of life, research has consistently shown that mood is related to *quality* of life. As Cheri Register wrote in *The Chronic Illness Experience: Embracing the Imperfect Life*, "How well people manage lives marked by illness depends not on the nature of the illness but on the strength of their conviction that life is worth living no matter what complications are imposed on it." This thought summarizes what many people who have been diagnosed with cancer know: that this disease doesn't define one's life but only complicates it. Sometimes your mood may be low despite healing well. If you have a persistent mood disturbance, such as depression, your quality of life will be significantly diminished. It does seem to be true that people who report that they have a good quality of life are more likely to follow their medical treatment plans. The bottom line is that *your emotional health is important for its own sake, but it is also important in your quest to physically heal.*

If you have a wonderful prognosis and your future looks bright, you may still feel sad and worried or even uncontrollably anxious and depressed. If you have a more advanced stage of cancer, a particularly difficult cancer to treat, or an incurable type of cancer, you may have the same emotional response—but with the treatments available today you may well have a long life. Still, there is no doubt that cancer is a heavy emotional burden to live with.

When something bad happens to people, they need to grieve. The well-known psychiatrist Elisabeth Kübler-Ross taught us that lesson, describing stages of grief that usually follow a certain order. It isn't necessary to go through all of the stages of grief or to grieve in the order that Kübler-Ross outlined, but it is important to grieve. If you have been diagnosed with cancer, grief is a normal and arguably an essential reaction. These are Kübler-Ross's five stages of grief:

Stage 1: Denial and isolation
Stage 2: Anger
Stage 3: Bargaining
Stage 4: Depression
Stage 5: Acceptance

You may be wondering where "hope" comes in. Kübler-Ross notes that hope is found within all of the stages. Hope is present almost always, though there may be times when you feel more or less hopeful. This variation, of course, is normal. Feeling consistently hopeless is a cardinal sign of more serious depression. Table 11.1 compares grief and depression symptoms.

There is no "right way" to feel about a cancer diagnosis. I once asked my father-in-law, who was diagnosed with thyroid cancer as a young man, whether he was scared at the time. Our conversation was decades after the incident, but he told me that he had not been particularly worried—he trusted his doctors implicitly. His response was not surprising,

Table 11.1. Symptoms of Grief and Symptoms of Depression	
Grief	*Depression*
Sleep disturbances, changes in appetite, decreased ability to concentrate, less interest in social activities, alterations in usual behavior patterns (for example, more irritable or angry)	Symptoms similar to those of grief but also may feel hopeless, helpless, worthless, and guilty and in some instances may have thoughts of suicide
Generally waxes and wanes and the person vacillates between feeling hopeful and sad; still able to enjoy activities	Constant feelings of intense sadness that affect most or all aspects of life; unable to enjoy activities

coming from a war veteran who was quite stoic and relatively unflappable.

Undoubtedly, we all handle things in our own way. Many people will go through most or all of the stages of grief that Kübler-Ross described. Other reactions may include the following:

Shock. Most people fear, but don't anticipate, a cancer diagnosis. Almost everyone goes through a period of shock during the initial crisis phase. Generally the shock wears off as time passes and as one becomes more educated about the specifics of the diagnosis.

Anger. Anger is a common reaction and a completely normal response to a life-altering situation. But uncontrolled anger is a dangerous emotion that can be detrimental to your health and to the health of those you love. As Aristotle noted, "Anyone can become angry. That is easy. But to be angry with the right person, to the right degree, at the right time, for the right purpose and in the right way—that is not easy."

Fear. Fear can take many forms and is not always about facing one's own mortality. Other issues can include the fear of the bills that will accumulate, the fear of being abandoned, and the fear of suffering from pain.

One of my friends went through breast cancer treatment at the same time I did. When she was initially diagnosed, her doctors gave her information about her prognosis, but all she heard was that she did not have the earliest stage; therefore, she would not have the best possible chance of recovery. She took in the information they told her and converted it in her mind into a terrible future, which wasn't accurate. She once told me, "When I heard my prognosis, it was like having a knife to my throat." Several months after her treatment ended, she asked her oncologist again about her prognosis. This time, though the information was essentially the same, she was amazed at what a good prognosis she really had once she got over the fear of a diagnosis of cancer that was not in the very earliest stage.

With cancer, the fear of facing your own mortality is extremely powerful. Getting the right information about your diagnosis and then doing what you need to do to treat your illness can help to lessen your fear. Keep in mind that it is fine to ask the same questions over and over again. It is difficult to take in all of the necessary information at the beginning.

Guilt. Probably every person diagnosed with cancer has thought, "What did I do wrong?" Maybe there is something that you can point to, but often the reasons for developing cancer elude us. No matter what you did or didn't do (diet, exercise, smoking, drinking, etc.), remember that no one "deserves" to get cancer. Moreover, most of us would admit that we could lead a more perfect life in terms of preventing illness. Being perfect isn't possible, though. We are human beings and capable of amazing accomplishments—but not perfection. If you feel guilty, for whatever reason, work through the feeling by talking to your doctors and others you trust.

Distress. Distress is a common symptom and may affect you at various times throughout cancer treatment and long afterward.

Anxiety. Often anxiety in cancer survivors stems from uncertainty about the future and is included in the other reactions mentioned in this section. For example, feeling a loss of control can lead to intense anxiety. So can overwhelming grief or guilt or feeling as though the burdens are insurmountable. Some worry is normal. But when anxious feelings begin to interfere with your thoughts repeatedly and your ability to cope and heal is affected, then you may want to get some professional help. (See Table 11.2 for symptoms of anxiety that may benefit from medical intervention.) There are two things that I always tell my anxious patients. The first is that anxious people are "quality" people.

Table 11.2. Symptoms of Anxiety	
Feeling tense or nervous	Having a stomachache
Feeling jittery or jumpy	Feeling light-headed or dizzy
Having difficulty relaxing	Having difficulty sleeping
Feeling fatigued	Feeling "on edge"
Having muscle aches	Feeling terrified without apparent
Feeling restless	reason
Feeling apprehensive	Anticipating impending doom
Feeling fearful or anticipating	Feeling short of breath
misfortune	Experiencing a choking or
Feeling sweaty or having clammy	smothering sensation
hands	Feeling faint
Feeling chest palpitations or heart	Trembling or shaking
racing	

By and large, anxious individuals are good people who lead meaningful lives. The second is that if there is one word that will calm your anxiety it is *acceptance*. Accepting what you must will soothe your worry.

You may find that at times you are experiencing again, though hopefully much more briefly, the same kinds of emotions you did when you were initially diagnosed. Everyone who has faced cancer has had her or his emotional baseline temporarily altered. Even if you think you are at your usual mood level, it is not uncommon—nor will it harm you—to have feelings of distress, worry, fear, grief, anxiety, and so on, resurface occasionally.

MOOD AND RECOVERY

Persistent symptoms associated with clinical depression, uncontrolled anxiety, or some other mood disorder might diminish your ability to physically heal from cancer treatment. Both clinical depression, often called major depression, and uncontrolled anxiety are medical conditions that call for treatment with medications or psychological counseling or both. There are many reasons that these conditions need to be treated, but here are the most important ones:

Both anxiety and depression can have a deleterious effect on sleep, which is necessary for optimal healing.

They are associated with increased levels of perceived pain, which can interfere with physical activity such as exercise.

They may hamper people's ability to make good treatment decisions.

They may impede their ability to adhere to a treatment plan.

Also, both major depression and uncontrolled anxiety are strongly related to a reduced quality of life, and the quality of one's life is extremely important, regardless of whatever else is happening. (See Tables 11.2 and 11.3 for symptoms of anxiety and depression.)

Depression is not unusual among those who are dealing with cancer and its aftereffects. Although someone can become depressed or anxious at any time after a cancer diagnosis, there seem to be times when people are particularly vulnerable. An obvious time is at the initial cancer diagnosis. But did you know that many people experience emotional setbacks when their cancer treatments end? It is ironic that the day that every cancer survivor looks forward to—the time when treatment will stop and they can resume their lives—can also mark the beginning of new emotional problems.

Several factors might contribute to an increase in emotional distress during the recovery phase. One is that the posttreatment care of can-

Table 11.3. Symptoms of Depression	
Losing interest in usual activities and pastimes	Sleeping too much
Feeling irritable	Feeling agitated or restless
Crying frequently	Feeling unusually fatigued
Feeling sad	Having difficulty concentrating
Feeling hopeless	Having difficulty making decisions
Having a poor appetite or significant weight loss	Feeling self-critical
	Feeling excessively guilty
Having an increased appetite or significant weight gain	Feeling worthless
	Having recurrent thoughts of dying or suicidal thoughts
Sleeping poorly	

cer patients usually is much less intense than the treatment phase. This means that one's interaction with reassuring healthcare providers is significantly reduced. Once you finish treatment, the next doctor's appointment might be weeks or months away. Many cancer patients describe feeling "cut loose" or "on their own" at this juncture.

Another reason mood disorders might become a problem during the posttreatment phase is that during active therapy people feel as though they are "doing something" to get rid of the cancer. After treatment there is more of a "watch and wait" plan. Although I didn't become clinically depressed after I stopped chemotherapy, I did feel let down and had a strong desire to be proactive about my health. I was not comfortable with just watching and waiting. That is why I decided to take the steps that I talk about in this book. End-of-treatment emotional distress may or may not result in clinical depression, but it is a well-known phenomenon among cancer survivors and is important to consider as you begin to rebuild your life. Posttraumatic stress disorder (PTSD), although not very common, has also been described in cancer survivors.

Finishing treatment and worrying about recurrence is not the only reason cancer survivors may suffer from emotional problems. For example, Fran Drescher, best known as the lead actress on the television sitcom *The Nanny*, was diagnosed with uterine cancer in 2000. After her uterus and ovaries were surgically removed (the only treatment she needed and chose to have) she began to think about the fact that she would never be able to bear a child. She was in her early 40s and had not wanted to have children up to this point, but having that option completely taken away bothered her. In her memoir, *Cancer Schmancer*, she wrote of what she was going through with her significant other: "John said we didn't need to have a biological baby to have a family. He's an extremely generous man and I love him for having said that. But, for a while there, I gotta admit, it was difficult to grasp the permanence of it all, and I found myself slipping into a depression."

Often a number of factors contribute simultaneously to a person's emotional crisis. One of my patients is a woman in her late 40s who is raising two teenage children. Several years ago she was diagnosed with breast cancer and underwent a lumpectomy and radiation treatment. More recently, she had a local recurrence of her cancer and opted for a mastectomy followed by reconstructive surgery and then chemotherapy. When I first saw her, there was no single reason for her depression. She was stressed over the teenage rebellion going on in her home. Sleep was difficult because of uncontrolled hot flashes, a result of premature menopause that was induced by the chemotherapy, and her shoulder hurt from the breast reconstruction. Friends and family members, including her husband, had been taxed by her initial cancer diagnosis, and now many of the members of her original support system were not able to be as helpful as they had been in the past. She wept in my office and told me, "One cancer diagnosis is bad enough, but two is just overwhelming!"

HOW PHYSICAL CHANGES CAN AFFECT EMOTIONS

Increasingly we are finding that mood disturbances, such as depression and anxiety, are largely due to chemical imbalances in the brain. Read this as *it's not your fault if you are experiencing symptoms of a mood disorder*. Hormones such as those associated with the thyroid gland or sex hormones such as estrogen and testosterone may be affected by cancer treatment for a number of reasons. Sometimes these hormones help to stimulate the growth of tumors and need to be suppressed intentionally as a means of treatment, while other times their levels drop simply as a side effect of other cancer treatment. Neurotransmitters like serotonin and norepinephrine may also be affected by cancer treatment for reasons that we don't clearly understand. Imbalances in hormones or neurotransmitters can lead to anxiety and depression. That is why antidepressant medications (also often used to treat anxiety) are so effective. Many of the antidepressant medications work by regulating serotonin and norepinephrine levels in the brain. You may have heard of the abbreviation SSRI, which stands for selective serotonin reuptake inhibitor—a relatively new class of antidepressant medications. Some of these drugs have names you might be familiar with: Paxil, Prozac, and Zoloft. A newer class of antidepressants is SNRIs (serotonin norepinephrine reuptake inhibitors), which include Effexor. These antidepressants are often very effective and improve emotional imbalances in most of the patients who try them. Table 11.4 provides a more detailed list of the subclasses of antidepressant medications.

Table 11.4. Antidepressant Medications

Selective Serotonin Reuptake Inhibitors (SSRIs)
   Action: Increase serotonin levels in the brain
   Drugs: Celexa (citalopram), Lexapro (escitalopram), Paxil (paroxetine),
      Prozac (fluoxetine), Zoloft (sertraline)
   Notable Side Effects: Nausea and stomach upset, agitation, difficulty
      sleeping, headache, decreased libido, and other sexual dysfunction
      (problems with erections, etc.). Rarely there are associated suicidal
      thoughts.

Serotonin Norepinephrine Reuptake Inhibitors (SNRIs)
   Action: Increase serotonin and norepinephrine levels in the brain
   Drugs: Cymbalta (duloxetine), Effexor (venlafaxine)
   Notable Side Effects: Nausea and stomach upset, sedation, dry mouth,
      tremors, and headache

Norepinephrine Dopamine Reuptake Inhibitors (NDRIs)
   Action: Increase serotonin and dopamine levels in the brain
   Drug: Wellbutrin (bupropion)
   Notable Side Effects: Agitation, weight loss, insomnia, elevated blood
      pressure, and liver toxicity. Patients with a history of seizures or an-
      orexia or bulimia should not take Wellbutrin. Also, Wellbutrin has the
      same active ingredient (bupropion) as is present in the antismoking
      medication Zyban, so they usually should not be taken together.

Noradrenergic Specific Serotonergic Antidepressants (NaSSAs)
   Action: Enhance norepinephrine and serotonin activity in the brain
   Drug: Remeron (mirtazapine)
   Notable Side Effects: dizziness, weight gain, lethargy, and liver toxicity

Serotonin Antagonist Reuptake Inhibitors (SARIs)
   Action: Increase serotonin levels in the brain
   Drugs: Desyrel (trazodone), Serzone (nefazodone)
   Notable Side Effects: Nausea and stomach upset, sedation, headache,
      dizziness. Desyrel is rarely associated with sustained and painful
      erection in men.

Tricyclic Antidepressants
   Action: Increase serotonin and norepinephrine levels in the brain
   Drugs: Anafranil (clomipramine), Elavil (amitryptiline), Norpramin
      (desipramine), Pamelor (nortryptiline), Sinequan (doxepin), Tofranil
      (imipramine)
   Notable Side Effects: Sedation, dry mouth, weight gain, and dizziness.
      Rarely associated with cardiac conduction delays (arrhythmias).

Only those mood problems that are persistent and disabling need to be treated with medication. By disabling, I mean that they interfere with your ability to function the way you would like to or the way you normally do. Prescription antidepressants are extremely helpful to some cancer survivors, but there are also other options to help stabilize or improve your mood.

WORKING TOWARD EMOTIONAL BALANCE

If you think you have symptoms of anxiety or depression, you should talk to your doctor about how you are feeling. Improving your emotional health will not only enhance your quality of life, but it will also help you to physically heal. One way your doctor can help is to consider the physical reasons behind your emotional problems. The more common physical factors are listed in Table 11.5. Just recognizing your symptoms and having a frank discussion with either your primary care physician or your oncologist is the first hurdle.

Your doctor will likely want to review the medications that you are taking. There are many prescription drugs that can contribute to emotional problems. Keep in mind that if you are on a medication that may have some unintended psychological side effects, your doctor might want you to stay on this drug because it treats other health concerns. Or there may be alternative treatments to try. I always recommend having this discussion with your physician rather than abruptly going off prescription medications. Avoid "self-medicating" with alcohol or other substances. Alcohol is a depressant, and although sometimes individuals use it to help relieve feelings of anxiety and frustration, it almost always has the opposite effect, particularly when used regularly. St. John's

Table 11.5. Physical Factors That Can Contribute to Emotional Problems	
Sex hormone imbalances	Adrenal gland problems
Neurotransmitter imbalances	Thyroid dysfunction
High calcium levels	Sodium or potassium imbalances
Anemia	Medication side effects
Nutritional deficiencies	Uncontrolled pain
Poor sleep	Neurological or musculoskeletal problems

wort is another product that people often use to help with their moods. Because of the many interactions of this compound with prescription medications, if you are taking St. John's wort, I recommend that you discuss it with your doctor.

You should also talk to your doctor about your sleep habits. Poor or fragmented sleep has been associated with a higher incidence of depression. If you are having issues related to either the cancer itself or the treatment (pain, hormonal imbalances, etc.), your doctor might want to treat these problems in order to improve your sleep and potentially help with your mood as well. Similarly, symptoms that occur during your waking hours, such as pain, may wear you down and cause you to feel more worried or sad. Pain, too, can usually be treated effectively. The bottom line is that if you are experiencing symptoms of emotional distress, think about what factors might be related to it and talk to your doctor about how he or she can help (see Table 11.6 for a list of concerns to discuss with your doctor).

You may be pleasantly surprised—your discussion with your doctor may lead to a relatively easy fix (such as improving your sleep or relieving your pain). Since depression and anxiety are typically due to chemical imbalances in the brain, your physician might suggest medications to improve your mood. Or there may not be a clear reason for your emotional symptoms, and your doctor may suggest counseling, cognitive behavioral therapy, meditation, guided imagery, trying an antidepressant, or a combination of these. Because emotional issues are so common in cancer patients, the majority of oncology treatment centers have a mental health component, although often such services are not available to patients unless they specifically request them. You should work with your physician to consider all of the factors that might be contributing to your symptoms and learn what type of treatment will help.

MENTAL HEALTH PROFESSIONALS

The mood disturbances that cancer survivors experience may in some cases be underdiagnosed and undertreated because both patients and healthcare workers often believe that it is normal to experience symptoms of depression or anxiety when one has been diagnosed with cancer. And often people's changes in baseline mood, appetite, or sleep

Table 11.6. What to Talk to Your Doctor About
Any anxious or depressive symptoms you are having that are listed in Tables 11.2 and 11.3
Any problems relating to sleeping well
Neurological or musculoskeletal problems
Persistent pain
Unusual or persistent fatigue
Difficulty with exercise
Medications and supplements you are taking
Whether you might have a hormonal, nutritional, or other chemical imbalance

patterns are minor or short lived. Persistent mood disturbances that result in clinical depression occur in probably less than 10 percent of cancer patients. There is a spectrum of mood problems that includes normal mood fluctuations, minor disturbances in mood that are outside the realm of normal but not necessarily pathologic, and more serious mood problems that are diagnosable. Recognizing that mood problems follow a spectrum, I developed a project at Harvard Medical School called *The Almost Effect*. (This is similar to physical problems such as blood pressure that may be normal, a little bit high, or quite high and diagnosed as hypertension.) The Almost Effect consists of a series of books on mental health conditions that don't quite reach the threshold for diagnosis. For example, two of the books in the series are *Almost Depressed* and *Almost Anxious*. You can learn more about The Almost Effect at www.TheAlmostEffect.com.

The statistics on mood disorders vary widely; however, reports suggest that as many as one-third of cancer patients may at some point express emotional concerns that warrant a workup. Therefore, while it is normal to feel sad, worried, or angry at times after being diagnosed with cancer, both patients and healthcare professionals need to recognize the symptoms of a more serious and persistent mood disturbance such as clinical depression or an anxiety disorder.

In oncology, mental health professionals (psychiatrists, clinical social workers, and psychologists), who focus on helping cancer patients recover emotionally, are almost always part of the healthcare team. Very often clergy participate as well. In the rehabilitation model of care, the model that I am trained in, there is also an important focus on what we sometimes call "adjustment to a disability or serious illness." This, of course, is the emotional component of recovery. Physicians in my specialty (physiatrists) are also well educated about the physical consequences of emotional health. That is why physiatrists by and large place great importance on the psychological well-being of their patients. Mental health professionals are part of the team of healthcare professionals who participate in the care of inpatient rehabilitation patients and are usually available in the outpatient setting as well. At many centers, there is an oncology social worker or psychologist who is dedicated to helping cancer survivors with both emotional and physical recovery goals.

Your primary care physician or oncologist may be the one to initiate treatment with an antidepressant medication or other interventions to help you during this stressful time. Most doctors are also able to provide referrals to mental health professionals who specialize in treating people with serious illnesses. You don't necessarily need to go to a psychiatrist, psychologist, or clinical social worker who treats only cancer patients, but the more experience the person has in oncology, the better informed she or he will be about what you are going through.

Although some psychiatrists continue to counsel patients, the current trend in medicine is for them to focus on starting and adjusting medications that treat mental health conditions. Psychologists and clinical social workers, who are not licensed to prescribe medications, perform counseling. These professionals can also be extremely skilled at teaching patients cognitive strategies to help with relaxation and stress reduction, such as meditation, biofeedback, and imagery. Some counselors, especially those who work closely with oncologists, can also provide information about a particular medical condition to help put things in perspective.

Treatment for emotional issues that are brought on by living with a cancer diagnosis is often effective and frequently entails low doses of antidepressant medications for several months and perhaps just a few visits with a mental health professional to assist with coping. Of course, the extent of the emotional issues can be affected by one's prognosis

Table 11.7. Symptoms of Posttraumatic Stress Disorder	
Mental flashbacks	Difficulty with concentration
Being startled by loud noises	Nightmares
Anxiety or depression	Irritability
Poor sleep	Anger

and by any pre-existing psychological issues such as a history of depression, substance abuse, childhood abuse, or PTSD (the latter occurs in a small percentage of cancer patients after they are diagnosed; see Table 11.7 for a list of symptoms). In such cases, therapy aimed at improving mental health might become more involved.

As I mentioned, both anxious and depressive symptoms are often temporary and caused by the extreme stress of a cancer diagnosis. A temporary mood disturbance may not require the use of antidepressant medications or counseling, but if you have symptoms that persist beyond a few weeks, consider seeking professional help. And if you have very severe symptoms such as an inability to sleep, significant loss of appetite, or thoughts of suicide, you should talk to your doctor right away. *A good rule to follow if you are experiencing symptoms of anxiety or depression is that you need professional help when your mood is interfering on a daily basis with either your quality of life or your ability to physically recover from cancer treatment.*

WHAT YOU CAN TRY ON YOUR OWN

Regardless of whether you seek out other treatment for your emotional well-being, there are strategies that you can use to help yourself. You may want to keep a journal; see the box on pages 193 and 194, where I describe how to begin. Table 11.8 lists some other suggestions that have been helpful to cancer survivors. Also refer to the other chapters in this book; they cover many of the topics listed in Table 11.8 in more depth. For example, in chapter 7 I discuss the enormous health benefits of exercise during the recovery period. One of the important and widely recognized side effects of regular cardiovascular exercise is an improvement in mood. Regular exercise can be a powerful antidote to a mood disturbance by releasing chemicals in your brain. The purely chemical result of exercise, endorphin release, is good for your emotions, but so are other outcomes, such as the boost to your self-esteem when you relearn to physically challenge yourself and trust your body again. If you have physical problems, ask your doctor about cancer prehabilitation and rehabilitation. Regardless of whether you have obvious physical impairments, you may still want to begin with formal exercise instruction from a physical therapist who is trained in cancer rehabilitation.

In chapter 13 I talk about how people with good support systems have a lower incidence of depression and a better quality of life. Reach out to your trusted friends, family members, or clergy who can be good listeners and provide you with the nurturing that you need during this time. Let your feelings out with someone you feel safe with. Communicating with your loved ones is an essential part of improving your psychological health and will also help you maintain good relationships

Table 11.8. Practical Things You Can Do to Improve Your Mood

Limit or avoid alcohol

Eat a well-rounded diet that is low in fat and high in fruits and vegetables

Get proper rest

Share your feelings with trusted family members, friends, or clergy

Consider joining a support group or contact some of the resources in the appendix for support

Exercise regularly

Practice meditating or imagery to help yourself relax

Commune with nature

Pray

Consider trying acupuncture

Consider having a massage or a manicure

Educate yourself about your diagnosis and how you can best help yourself

Keep a journal

Preserve routines that are comforting

Surround yourself with "feel-good" media (books, television, and movies)

Continue hobbies that give you pleasure

Set limits with family, friends, and coworkers about what you are able to do

Avoid self-blame

Get together with friends

Engage in a favorite hobby

Starting a Journal

If you have never written in a journal, now might be a good time to start. Studies show that people who commit their deepest emotions to paper receive significant emotional health benefits. Even the national media have caught on to the potential health benefits of keeping a journal. *Newsweek* magazine published an article titled "Pen, Paper, Power!" In this piece journalist Claudia Kolb wrote, "Confessional writing has been around at least since the Renaissance, but new research suggests that it's far more therapeutic than anyone ever knew. Since the mid-1980s, studies have found that people who write about their most upsetting experiences not only feel better but visit doctors less often and even have stronger immune responses."

Kathryn Koob was one of the Americans who was held hostage for over a year during the Carter administration's crisis with Iran. During this time she kept a journal on the backs of envelopes. She later said, "My journal helped me remember my reactions and some things I had read. It also reminded me of things I wanted to think about more deeply and helped me crystallize my thinking."

Myra Schneider, a poet who wrote a book called *Writing My Way through Cancer,* recounts her own experiences with breast cancer and offers advice about how writing can help. At one point in her recovery, Myra describes emotions that many cancer survivors experience: "While I was recuperating from the operation and undergoing treatment I frequently felt frightened or upset but rarely depressed. I not only braced myself to go through the ordeal, I clung like a leech to everything life-giving and positive. Now, however, I often feel depressed—as if everything's impossibly hard, as if health and ordinary living are forever out of reach. Any problems throw me completely." Two days later she wrote, "It's dawned on me that this feeling of being completely overwhelmed is to be expected and that if I keep blaming myself for managing badly I'm simply giving myself another problem."

Kathryn Koob and Myra Schneider both turned to writing as a way to deal with the intense emotional impact of their very different life-threatening ordeals. If you are inclined to try keeping a journal, you may find it helpful in that you can express your greatest fears in the privacy of its pages. Also, in many people's experience, the act of writing something down somehow gives the thought less power over them. Writing may help "crystallize" your thoughts and motivate you in your recovery or help direct your future medical care, employment decisions, and participating with friends and loved ones.

Psychology professor James Pennebaker is a researcher in the field of expressive writing and its health benefits. In his book *Writing to Heal,* he tells readers that they may feel sad immediately after writing about something traumatic: "Emotional writing can be likened to seeing a sad movie; afterward you feel sadder but wiser. . . . Expressive writing may make you sad for a brief time after doing it, but the long-term effects are surely worth the momentary sadness." Some of the long-term effects include reduced depression and anxiety and a generally improved mood.

As you begin keeping a journal, decide where you want to keep your record. Some people prefer to use the computer, while others like to write in a special book. If you use the computer, be sure to back up your journal so that you don't lose it if your computer crashes. If you are worried about privacy, you can use password protection to keep the information confidential. If you want a hard copy, you can print the pages and place them in a folder next to your computer.

When writing for yourself, put down whatever comes to mind. You do not need to follow any of the usual writing rules (proper spelling and grammar, a topic sentence at the beginning of each paragraph, etc.). You can skip from one idea to the next without transitions. You can write in incomplete sentences, use abbreviations, and illustrate as desired. If you can't find a quiet place to write or you don't have much time, it doesn't matter. You can write in your journal for just a couple of minutes in the midst of great commotion. There are no rules, so there is no way for you to make a mistake or do the job incorrectly. Whatever you write, however you write it, is fine.

with people who support you. In addition, you may benefit from joining a support group made up of people who are suffering with the same or a similar illness.

As you think about your own situation, recognize that you need to be good to yourself. Excessively worrying about your mood is counterproductive. Instead, step out of the situation for a moment and look at yourself as though you were a loved one. What would you advise that loved one to do? Would you encourage him or her to get professional help, knowing that it might aid with physical as well as emotional recovery? Whether you decide to seek assistance for your emotional health, remember that there are many approaches that you can take other than psychological counseling or taking an antidepressant medication. Just as you carefully considered the options for treating your cancer, I encourage you to consider your emotional health and how it can impact your recovery.

References

H. Jordan, *No Such Thing as a Bad Day* (New York: Simon and Schuster, 2000).

Institute of Medicine, *Cancer Care for the Whole Patient: Meeting Psychosocial Health Needs* (Washington, DC: National Academies Press, 2007).

E. Banks, J. E. Byles, R. E. Gibson, B. Rodgers, I. K. Latz, I. A. Robinson, et al., "Is Psychological Distress in People Living with Cancer Related to the Fact of Diagnosis, Current Treatment or Level of Disability? Findings from a Large Australian Study," supplement, *Medical Journal of Australia* 193, no. 5 (2010): S62–S67.

K. E. Weaver, L. P. Forsythe, B. B. Reeve, C. M. Alfano, J. L. Rodriguez, S. A. Sabatino, N. A. Hawkins, and J. H. Rowland, "Mental and Physical Health-Related Quality of Life among U.S. Cancer Survivors: Population Estimates from the 2010 National Health Interview Survey," *Cancer Epidemiology, Biomarkers & Prevention* 21, no. 11 (November 2012): 2108–17.

J. Holland, *The Human Side of Cancer: Living with Hope, Coping with Uncertainty* (New York: HarperCollins, 2000), pp. 4, 14.

C. Register, *The Chronic Illness Experience: Embracing the Imperfect Life* (Center City, MN: Hazelden, 1989), p. xxii.

J. K. Rustad, D. David, and M. B. Currier, "Cancer and Post-traumatic Stress Disorder: Diagnosis, Pathogenesis and Treatment Considerations," *Palliative & Supportive Care* 10, no. 3 (September 2012): 213–23.

Luana Marques with Eric Metcalf, *Almost Anxious* (Center City, MN: Hazelden, 2013).

Jefferson Prince and Shelley Carson, *Almost Depressed* (Center City, MN: Hazelden, 2013).

F. Drescher, *Cancer Schmancer* (New York: Warner Books, 2002), p. 184.

C. Kolb, "Pen, Paper, Power!" *Newsweek*, April 26, 1999.

M. Schneider, *Writing My Way through Cancer* (London: Jessica Kingsley, 2003), pp. 130–31.

J. W. Pennebaker, *Writing to Heal* (Oakland, CA: New Harbinger, 2004), p. 8.

CHAPTER 12

TAP INTO YOUR
SPIRITUALITY

One morning, about a year after I was diagnosed with breast cancer, I was driving somewhere with my then 12-year-old son, and I asked him, "Do you ever get worried about my having had cancer?" As I looked in the rear view mirror at this half boy-half man, he said somewhat nonchalantly, "No. I don't really think about it." I was a bit surprised but just chalked it up to the fact that he was a child, still very self-absorbed. We were both quiet for a few minutes and then he spoke again, "But I pray for you every night." This confession brought me to tears. What an amazing gift, I thought. *My son prays for me every night.* As I surreptitiously wiped my eyes, I realized that this was the perfect opportunity to talk to my eldest child about spirituality and illness. That morning we discussed many of the things that I have included in this chapter.

Some people might find a chapter on spirituality and illness in a book such as this off-putting. I debated whether to include it. However, since it has been a topic of research, I decided that I should share with interested readers what we know about how spirituality, religion, and prayer may influence health and healing. My intention is not to encourage or discourage any specific religious beliefs or spiritual ideology. I have a deep respect for the sanctity of a person's own beliefs. My goal here is simply to give you access to what healthcare professionals know about the relevance of spirituality to physical health.

Some Definitions

The following definitions are offered as a framework for discussion. I'll define *spirituality* as those things that relate to one's spirit. Spirituality may be used in a religious or a nonreligious context. Often people who are not religious nevertheless see themselves as spiritual beings and consider nature to be a force to connect with their feelings of spirituality. A dictionary definition of *spirit* is "an animating or vital principle held to give life to physical organisms." It can also be defined as "a special attitude or frame of mind." So, spirituality in the physical healing context can be simply a state of mind that is focused on a source of external energy such as nature or God. *Religion*, while overlapping with spirituality, is a more formal concept that includes codes of behavior and rules of conduct. According to Harold Koenig, a leading authority in the science of spirituality, "Religion involves beliefs about the transcendent, as well as private or communal practices and rituals that reflect devotion or commitment to those beliefs." *Faith* is defined as a belief in something for which there is no proof.

Prayer is generally thought of in a religious context, but it can be a nonreligious endeavor and associated with the nonreligious aspects of spirituality. In her book *How to Pray without Being Religious*, psychologist Janell Moon writes, "Webster's New World Dictionary defines prayer as 'the act or practice of praying, to beg, to implore or beseech, implore, to ask earnestly; make supplication as to a deity; to God, a god, as by reciting certain set formulas.' I propose that we expand the definition of prayer to include praying to our spirit as a source of life energy." So, for the purposes of this discussion, prayer, which can include meditation and other nonreligious practices, is the method that one uses to connect to one's energy source. Although some scholars make a clear delineation between prayer and meditation, for this chapter, I'll include them in one general category. Formal religion may or may not be a part of an individual's spiritual life. Moreover, these definitions are inclusive; practically anyone, even those who are nonbelievers, may be able to tap into spiritual resources as a method of healing.

Throughout history, religious practices and rituals have been an intrinsic part of healing. In fact, they were often the only methods of healing—particularly when there were few medical remedies that worked. Much of the current literature in psychoneuroimmunology has focused on modern-day religious practices (for example, regularly attending church) and how they impact health.

Although much of the research to date has focused on religious practices, according to numerous studies, Americans are becoming less religious than they were in the past. The majority of people living in the United States continue to report that they are religious, however, and, of those who don't identify with a specific religion, many still consider themselves spiritual. For example, a survey conducted by Pew Research found that 65 percent of the people surveyed said they were religious and 18 percent said they were spiritual only (and not religious).

People worldwide often report that spirituality or religious beliefs and activities provide them with comfort and reduce stress when they are facing illness. Many studies have reported less anxiety, depression, and fear among people facing illness who embraced religion. It's no surprise that individuals who are religious tend to have larger support systems, in part because religion fosters the gathering of groups. Regular churchgoers have been shown in some studies to live longer. A possible reason is that the religious culture tends to discourage smoking and drinking, encourage exercise, and foster social connections—all of which tend to help people to have longer lives. In response to the interest in and potential positive health effects of existential beliefs, more than half of all U.S. medical schools now offer courses in spirituality and healing.

Religiousness has been associated with reduced suicide, divorce, and substance abuse rates and with better coping with and acceptance of chronic illness, prolonged survival in the frail elderly, and speedier rehabilitation after surgery. *But what about cancer?* In a medical journal article titled "Spirituality and Religion in Oncology," the authors reviewed the current scientific literature on this topic and found that spiritual well-being correlated positively with better quality of life or psychosocial functioning in studies that have been done with prostate, breast, and gynecologic cancer survivors. This doesn't mean that it's not helpful with other types of cancers—it's that these are the populations that have been studied the most. Better quality of life and psychosocial functioning has also been demonstrated in patients undergoing radiation therapy. Spirituality also seems to help alleviate some of the symptoms of anxiety and depression that are associated with cancer or its treatment.

Harold Koenig, MD, is the director of Duke University's Center for Spirituality, Theology and Health. He has published extensively on the intersection between spirituality and health—more than four hundred scientific articles and book chapters and more than forty books. More than a decade ago, his book *The Link between Religion and Health* described the relationship between religion and stress. For example, people who regularly attend church services have been shown to have reduced levels of stress. Reduced stress has been correlated with decreased cortisol levels and an increased number of natural killer cells, which help to search for and destroy cancer cells in the body. Whether religion can affect immune function is still not clear. It is within the realm of possibility, however—and perhaps more likely than not—that religion (or nonreligious spirituality) may impact health in a positive way, especially for cancer survivors. In a more recent scientific review titled "Religion, Spirituality, and Health: The Research and Clinical Implications," Dr. Koenig describes the many benefits of religiosity and spirituality. Table 12.1 lists some of the highlights from this review with a focus on how they may affect someone diagnosed with cancer.

Next, let's take a look at some historical issues relating to religion and health and discuss more about the field of psychoneuroimmunology that has emerged to legitimately study what benefits spirituality may have on healing.

PAST TRANSGRESSIONS AND THE EMERGENCE OF PSYCHONEUROIMMUNOLOGY

Although embracing a spiritual life has been shown to improve health in a variety of ways, a skeptical view of this notion is understandable. Historically, religion has sometimes been used as a cover to perform

Table 12.1. Possible Health Benefits of Spirituality or Religion

Research on the relationship between spirituality and religiosity as it pertains to *psychological* health suggests that spirituality or religiosity may help cancer survivors to:

Better cope with adversity

Experience more positive emotions

Have an increased sense of well-being or happiness

Be more optimistic or hopeful

Believe that they have meaning and a purpose in life

Enjoy higher self-esteem

Feel a stronger sense of control

Develop more positive character traits

Lower their stress levels

Decrease symptoms of anxiety or depression

Avoid substance abuse

Have more stable marriages or other partner relationships

Experience more social support and social capital

Research on the relationship between spirituality or religiosity as it pertains to *physical* health suggests that spirituality or religiosity may help cancer survivors to:

Be more active and increase exercise

Physically function at a higher level

Reduce pain or manage it more effectively

Improve diet and lower cholesterol levels

Avoid nicotine and other harmful substances

Improve cancer prognosis*

Source: H. G. Koenig. "Religion, Spirituality, and Health: The Research and Clinical Implications." *ISRN Psychiatry* 2012 (December 16, 2012).

*The studies to date suggest that there may be a positive correlation with cancer prognosis, but this could be due to factors such as increasing exercise, reducing stress, and improving one's diet.

truly heinous acts—some of which were purported as necessary to ensure the health of a particular community (even "ethnic cleansing" has been promoted as a public health issue). Today, religion is often considered antithetical to modern medicine because medicine is based in science and religion is not. Certainly one reason that doctors (and patients) often attempt to keep spirituality and science separate is that the history of nonscientific medicine is rife with tales of voodoo, witchcraft, and phony faith healers.

The Supreme Court in 1996 ruled in a case that had to do with prayer and faith healing. The *New York Times* ran an op-ed piece titled "The Power of Prayer, Denied" and began the article with the following information:

> When Thomas Jefferson described religious freedom as "the most inalienable and sacred of all human rights," he could not have imagined that the time would come when American citizens would be forced to pay ruinous damages for enforcing it. But that is the result of the Supreme Court's decision last week not to review the case of *McKown v. Lundman*. The decision let stand a Minnesota Court of Appeals ruling upholding an award of $1.5 million to the father of 11-year-old Ian Lundman, who died in 1989 after his mother, stepfather and two Christian Science practitioners tried to use prayer to heal his diabetes.

In another case reported in the *New York Times*, a couple was convicted of involuntary manslaughter and sentenced to at least two and a half years in prison for relying on prayer instead of medicine to treat their daughter's diabetes. Several years earlier, they had been put on probation when their son died of an ear infection that they didn't treat medically.

Dr. William Nolen, a physician, wrote about his experience with a widely publicized faith healer during the early 1970s. Dr. Nolen attended a service conducted by Katherine Kuhlman, a leading evangelical healer, who reported the names of twenty-five people who had been "miraculously healed." Dr. Nolen performed some follow-up interviews, including one of a woman with cancer of the spine who at Kuhlman's command had discarded her brace and run across the stage. The following day, her backbone collapsed and four months later she died.

In *The Faith Healers*, James Randi wrote about how in 1986 he helped to expose another infamous charlatan, Peter Popoff, on NBC's *Tonight Show* (popularly known then as the *Johnny Carson Show*). Randi showed Americans that during a nationally televised "healing" session,

Popoff's wife had transmitted to him information that he represented as supernaturally received. Accounts of such frauds and abuses have become common over the years, and so it is no wonder that there are many skeptics who doubt all things having to do with spirituality and religion.

Nevertheless, the medical literature is increasingly supportive of the legitimate role of spirituality in healing. After thousands of years of people's use of religion, prayer, and spirituality to heal, these matters have become an area of intense scientific study. This emerging field, *psychoneuroimmunology*, seeks to identify what components are helpful in healing. Koenig writes, "Although this area of research is only in its infancy, and the data do not show causation, the preliminary findings are provocative and consistent with the hypothesis that religious involvement may reduce stress and stress-induced neuroendocrine and immune changes." One research topic that I am following closely is the link between natural killer cell activity and stress (discussed in chapter 2). Since there are scientific ways to measure natural killer cell activity, stress-related physical responses, tumor growth, and so on, it is possible to legitimately study how spirituality and religion affect health and healing.

A Spiritual Crisis

A cancer diagnosis may bring about a spiritual crisis. Spirituality is often a central component of dealing with serious illness. Research shows that many cancer survivors face a spiritual crossroads and some are in crisis. This seems to be particularly true for people who are diagnosed with more advanced cancer, as they often report feeling abandoned by God. Many cancer survivors say that they want more help with their spiritual needs, and studies have demonstrated that patients believe attention to their spiritual concerns is an important part of cancer care by physicians and nurses. In one study, lung cancer patients and their caregivers reported that religious faith was the second-most important factor that influenced their treatment decisions—the first was what the oncologist recommended.

Although many cancer survivors face a spiritual crisis, studies also show that there is an opportunity for *posttraumatic growth*—meaning that many cancer survivors find that this traumatic experience helps them to change in positive ways. For example, in one study cancer survivors described examples of positive changes in their relationships, perceptions of their own self-worth, and life in general. The participants were also able to adopt some lifestyle changes such as exercise.

Patricia Sealy is a nurse who wrote an essay in a medical journal that focuses on spirituality and religion about being diagnosed with locally advanced breast cancer. She described both a crisis and post-traumatic growth. Her essay began with these words: "Coming face-to-face with death was a spiritual crisis." Patricia went on to write about how much she and her family suffered. Reflecting on her experience, she explained, "By the end of my grueling treatment, I realized survival meant I needed to redirect the tremendous energy I was using to ruminate about the painful past toward healing in the present. . . . I learned that physical, emotional, and spiritual healing can occur in the midst of chaos."

In my book, *What Helped Get Me Through: Cancer Survivors Share Wisdom and Hope*, I asked people to share how religion and spirituality helped them. Not surprisingly, many people wrote about how their cancer diagnosis put them in a crisis mode, and this affected their spiritual or religious beliefs in many ways. For some this included a spiritual crisis, and they felt as though they were somehow being abandoned or punished for past transgressions. For others, the diagnosis increased their connection to whatever belief system they previously had. Still others said that they were newly exploring spirituality. I was interested to see that even for those who said they were neither religious nor spiritual, they generally (though not always) appreciated the cards, prayers, and other sentiments from loved ones. These are some highlights from what they shared:

Spirituality did help me. It made my mind stronger by allowing me to concentrate on my fight. (non-Hodgkin lymphoma survivor)

I am not a religious person (I guess that's the scientist in me), but I do believe in a greater good that brings people together. Call it a Zen state or whatever, but finding some sort of inner peace can go a long way. (testicular cancer survivor)

I saw how much my parents hurt for me and how scared they were of losing me. Knowing that God loves me even more than they do, I knew He was with me every step of the way. I read scripture, sang, listened to Christian music, and prayed (and prayed, and prayed . . .). When I was suffering the most, I would imagine that my bed was the hand of God, I always felt better as I felt Him hold me up and carry me through the pain or sadness. (endometrial cancer survivor)

I am not a particularly religious person, but my family is and I did find it comforting when people told me that they were praying for me or that I was in their prayers. It was also comforting to receive little medals or prayer cards. (chronic myelogenous leukemia and kidney cancer survivor)

If one considers gratitude, love of the world to be spiritual thoughts—then, I guess I felt very spiritual. (breast cancer survivor)

I am a chaplain, and I am Catholic. Religion and spirituality are my lifelines. (colorectal cancer survivor)

I have had the good fortune to travel extensively and have lived overseas several times. The contact with other cultures has helped broaden my perspective on life. Drawing on spiritual insights from these varying cultures helped me deal with the emotional challenge of this disease. (prostate cancer survivor)

My Jewish faith gets me through all of life, and it did not desert me during cancer. (breast cancer survivor)

At first, I blamed God. I wondered, "Why me? What did I do to deserve this?" Then I realized that pity thinking was getting me nowhere. I started praying for healing, and I began eating healthier. (melanoma skin cancer survivor)

When I found out I was ill, I renewed my interest in the Buddhist philosophy, finding it very calming and reassuring. (lung cancer survivor)

Prayer, prayer, and more prayer. You have to believe in something or someone to help you get through the cancer ordeal. (ovarian cancer survivor)

PRAYER

Another of my colleagues who works in the field of oncology, Dr. Jerome Groopman (probably best known for his book *The Anatomy of Hope*), wrote in a journal article about one of his patients who had cancer. She told him, "Doctor, I'm frightened. I pray every day. I want you to pray for me." Dr. Groopman didn't know what to say. He explained, "None of the training I received in medical school, residency, fellowship, or practice had taught me how to respond to Anna. . . . [S]hould I cross the boundary from the purely professional to the personal and join her in prayer?" This dilemma, of how much doctors should encourage our patients in prayer and even pray with them, is on the minds of many physicians. Not long ago, I told a patient that I would pray for her, and she responded that this meant more to her than any of the medications or other treatments I had prescribed. So what did Dr. Groopman do? He continues:

> And so, unsure of where to fix the boundary between the professional and the personal, unsure what words were appropriate, I drew on the Talmudic custom of my ancestors and the pedagogical practice of my mentors and answered her question with a question.
> "What is the prayer you want?"
> "Pray for God to give my doctors wisdom," Anna said.
> To that, I silently echoed, "Amen."

Prayer is usually considered to be a method of connecting with God or another concept or person, although prayer can also have meaning in a nonreligious context. Intercessory prayer is praying for someone besides yourself. Although the medical literature documents significant potential positive health benefits that result from praying for yourself, the literature is less clear and somewhat contradictory about whether intercessory prayer works. Dr. Larry Dossey has long believed that prayer helps people to heal. In his book *Prayer Is Good Medicine*, he wrote about the widely held belief that prayer is simply reciting aloud words that have been handed down from generation to generation. Dossey is inclusive in his concept of prayer and how individuals, regardless of their faith or adherence to a specific religion, can incorporate it:

Jesus Christ and the founders of Christianity did not speak English. Neither were the founders of any other of the major world religions fluent in our tongue. And, what about gender? Many people who pray do not address a male image but rather address Goddess. . . . Millions reject any form of a personal god to whom prayers could be addressed. An example is Buddhism, which is not a theistic religion. Buddhists pray not to a personal deity but to the Universe. . . . In its simplest form, prayer *is an attitude of the heart*—a matter of *being*, not doing.

Prayer is a cornerstone of the Christian faith. The Bible says, "For surely I know the plans I have for you, says the Lord, plans for your welfare and not for harm, to give you a future with hope. Then when you call upon me and come and pray to me, I will hear you" (Jeremiah 29:11–14, New Revised Standard Version). Catholics use the rosary for prayer, whereas Protestants pray in other ways.

Moreover, prayer is an important part of most religions. For people of the Jewish faith it's called the *davening;* for Buddhists prayer involves *meditation;* for Muslims prayer is called *salat* and is performed five times each day. Prayer is also practiced in lesser-known faiths. For example, healing prayers in the traditional Navajo community can range from an hour-long prayer to a nine-day reciting of chants. The medicine men who guide the ceremonies are called *hatali*, or chanters. The Pennsylvania Dutch community combines practices they brought with them to the New World several hundred years ago with elements they learned from Native American medicine men. According to one article on the healing practices of the Pennsylvania Dutch, much of their prayer occurs in the form of pow-wows. Men and women, called *brauchers*, or pow-wowers, are trained for these ceremonies. They don't advertise their services, and generally they hold other types of employment. Pow-wowers are "highly trusted, ethical members of their community, and are sought out by community people when necessary."

Prayer is, above all, a personal attempt to connect. Particularly during cancer treatment, though, people may feel "spiritually dry." Mark Thibodeaux, a Jesuit priest, writes, "Many people have the mistaken notion that those who have a strong prayer life never have problems experiencing God's presence in prayer. But any long-term pray-er will tell you that it is not unusual to go through long periods without feeling anything at all in one's prayer."

Whether you feel spiritually dry or you prefer not to partake in a religious type of prayer, there are ways to pray that may appeal to you and help you to heal. Moon describes some ways to pray that are nontraditional. For example, she suggests writing out a prayer using your own words, walking in a labyrinth or some other lovely place, focusing on a part of nature such as a leaf, or taking a soulful shower. More traditional healing prayers are listed in Table 12.2.

Regardless of your spiritual orientation, consider what Dossey has to say about prayer in *Healing Beyond the Body*: "Margaret Mead, the noted anthropologist, once said, 'Prayer does not use any artificial energy, it doesn't burn up any fossil fuel, it doesn't pollute.' It has another attribute Mead didn't mention, which should be of interest to all health-care professionals: it apparently works."

MEDITATION

Meditation may be a form of prayer for some people. Others look at it as a separate entity. Meditation is a process whereby normal thoughts are suspended in favor of another focus. The point of meditation can vary depending on one's beliefs, but, from a medical point of view, it has the ability to (at least temporarily) lower a person's blood pressure and heart rate and reduce physical signs of stress (for example, muscle tension). One study done on mindfulness meditation in cancer patients found that this type of meditation decreased mood disturbances and stress symptoms in both men and women with a wide variety of types of cancer. Meditation also seems to be helpful with reducing pain and managing the symptoms better. There are many ways that people meditate; some forms of meditation with simple instructions are explained in Table 12.3.

Meditation may feel awkward at first. Most people report that it gets easier and that they feel better with practice, however. Many good resources (for example, books, CDs, DVDs, and online videos) can be purchased in bookstores to help you get started. Most cancer centers also offer information and lessons on meditation. Other resources for

Table 12.2. Prayers for Healing

Send me, O God, your healing, so that I may quickly recover from the illness that has come upon me. Sustain my spirit, relieve my pain and restore me to perfect health, happiness and strength. Grant unto my body your healing power so I may continue to be able to bear testimony to your everlasting mercy and love, for you, O Lord, art a faithful and merciful healer. (This nondenominational example was selected by the pastoral care staff at the Mount Zion Medical Center, which is affiliated with the University of California at San Francisco.)

Thus saith the Lord, the God of David thy father, I have heard thy prayer, I have seen thy tears; behold, I will heal thee. (2 Kings 20:5, King James Version)

Let me not pray to be sheltered from dangers,
but to be fearless in facing them.
Let me not beg for the stilling of my pain,
but for the heart to conquer it.
Let me not crave in anxious fear to be saved,
but for the patience to win my freedom. (Buddhist prayer)

Say unto them O Muhammad: For those who believe it is a guidance and a healing.
(Koran 41:44–51)

May the One who blessed our ancestors—
Sarah, Rebecca, Rachel, and Leah,
Abraham, Isaac, and Jacob,
bless and heal the one who is ill:
[name], daughter/son of [name].
May the Holy One, the fountain of blessings,
shower abundant mercies upon her/him,
fulfilling her dreams of healing,
strengthening her with the power of life.
Merciful One:
restore her,
heal her,
strengthen her,
enliven her.
Send her complete healing
from the heavenly realms,
a healing of body and
a healing of soul,
together with all who are ill,
soon, speedily, without delay;
and let us say:
Amen! (Mishaberach—a traditional Jewish prayer for the sick)

Table 12.3. Examples of Meditation Practices

Mindfulness

This type of meditation is advocated by Jon Kabat-Zinn, who describes it in this way: "Mindfulness is an ancient Buddhist practice which has profound relevance for our present-day lives. This relevance has nothing to do with Buddhism per se or with becoming a Buddhist, but it has everything to do with waking up and living in harmony with oneself and with the world. It has to do with examining who we are, with questioning our view of the world and our place in it, and with cultivating some appreciation for the fullness of each moment we are alive. Most of all, it has to do with being in touch." In his book *Wherever You Go There You Are*, Kabat-Zinn helps readers get started with this advice:

> TRY: Setting aside a time every day for just being. Five minutes would be fine, or ten or twenty or thirty if you want to venture that far. Sit down and watch the moments unfold, with no agenda other than to be fully present. Use the breath as an anchor to tether your attention to the present moment. Your thinking mind will drift here and there, depending on the currents and winds moving in the mind until, at some point, the anchor line grows taut and brings you back. This may happen a lot. Bring your attention back to the breath, in all its vividness, every time it wanders. Keep the posture erect but not stiff. Think of yourself as a mountain.*

Breath-Focused Meditation

This technique is often taught in childbirth classes and focuses on the process of breathing for relaxation. In *Active Wellness*, Gayle Reichler suggests trying to do it this way:

> TRY: Close your eyes and begin deep breathing through your nose, focusing on your breath as it travels in and out of your body. If it helps you maintain your focus, count to 3 as you inhale and then count to 4 as you exhale. At first, you may find yourself easily distracted by outside noises and by your own thoughts, random images, and feelings. Observe any thoughts, images, feelings, and distractions that come up during meditation, but try not to become "attached" to them. Picture them as clouds floating through your mind. Observe them calmly, but let them go and return to focusing on your breath. As you continue your meditation practice, you will find it easier to remain focused on your breath.†

---

*Jon Kabat-Zinn, *Wherever You Go There You Are: Mindfulness Meditation in Everyday Life* (New York: Hyperion, 1994), pp. 3, 105.
†Gayle Reichler, *Active Wellness* (New York: Time-Life Books, 1998), p. 198.

Table 12.3. *(continued)*

Visualization and Imagery

   To meditate in this way, one concentrates on (visualizes) a specific vision or event. The theory behind this method is that the mind is able to cure the body when visualized images evoke sensory memory, strong emotions, or fantasy. For example, one of my patients, who was a mother with young children at the time of her diagnosis (and is now a long-term cancer survivor), used this technique and repeatedly imagined herself in the future at her daughter's wedding. An image I particularly like is from a painted card that an artist friend and cancer survivor sent me. The card shows the image of a tree. If you look closely, you can see that the tree is also a woman. The two images are meshed together. On the back of the painting my friend wrote, "Strong as a tree—and reaching up—up to faith and surrounded by those who love her."

> TRY: Imagine that in front of you is an elevator. The door is open and you walk in. . . . Picture the number of the level your healing guide will be on, and push that button. Let the elevator descend slowly to that level. When the doors open, you will be at the place where you will meet your healing guide. The doors may open to your special place, your inner workshop; to an office; to a place outdoors; or to somewhere else. When the doors open, you will see, hear, or feel the presence of your healing guide. . . . Tell the guide that you have an illness or problem you want to work on. Ask if the guide will help you with this illness. Tell the guide that you will describe your illness; wait for a reply. To help you describe your illness, you can create a mental image of your body, either in the air or on a screen. Show the guide the areas of your body that you think are ill. . . . Try to visualize the area of your illness as clearly as possible. . . . Now ask your guide how you can heal this illness. Listen carefully to the reply.*

Transcendental Meditation

   This type of meditation involves focusing on a mantra (a sound, a word, or a phrase that is repeated over and over either out loud, as a chant, or silently). Transcendental meditation was brought to the world's attention in the 1970s by the Beatles, who practiced it.

*Michael Samuels, *Healing with the Mind's Eye* (Hoboken, NJ: Wiley, 2003), pp. 164–67.

mind-body healing, such as the Cancer Support Community, are listed in the appendix.

THE RELAXATION RESPONSE

Dr. Herbert Benson, a colleague of mine who is a cardiology professor at Harvard, is widely known for his work on stress and relaxation. In the 1970s he coined the term *relaxation response* to refer to the opposite of the stress response commonly known as *fight or flight*. In a stressful situation, the nervous system goes into overdrive and increases the heart rate, blood pressure, breathing rate, and blood supply to the muscles; these are ways to help the body respond to stress. The relaxation response, in contrast, works by encouraging the nervous system to have the opposite effect. In his book *The Relaxation Response*, Dr. Benson states the two essential steps to eliciting the relaxation response:

1. Repeat a word, sound, phrase, prayer, or muscular activity.
2. Passively disregard everyday thoughts that inevitably come to mind and return to your repetition.

He then explains how to perform the technique:

1. Pick a focus word, short phrase, or prayer that is firmly rooted in your belief system.
2. Sit quietly in a comfortable position.
3. Close your eyes.
4. Relax your muscles, progressing from your feet to your calves, thighs, abdomen, shoulders, head, and neck.
5. Breathe slowly and naturally, and, as you do, say your focus word, sound, phrase, or prayer silently to yourself as you exhale.
6. Assume a passive attitude. Don't worry about how well you're doing. When other thoughts come to mind, simply say to yourself, "Oh well," and gently return to your repetition.
7. Continue for 10–20 minutes.
8. Do not stand immediately. Continue sitting quietly for a minute or so, allowing other thoughts to return. Then open your eyes and sit for another minute before rising.

9. Practice the technique once or twice daily. Good times to do so are before breakfast and before dinner.

Doing What Works for You

American Lama Surya Das writes, "When we are recovering from loss of any kind, we need to find ways to reconnect with our basic sanity and essential, authentic selves; we need to find kind ways to heal and put ourselves back together again. . . . Chanting, mantras, prayers, and meditation practice can be very healing and nurturing. Yoga and spiritual exercise, like physical exercise, is a beautiful way of being good to yourself."

Lynn Eib was diagnosed with advanced colon cancer at the age of 36. Having survived her cancer, she now works as a cancer patient advocate and is the author of *When God and Cancer Meet*. She writes, "The heart of a cancer survivor needs to find the right attitude. . . . The mind of a cancer survivor needs to find peace. . . . Finally, the soul of a cancer survivor needs to find hope." Whatever you decide to do will be right for you. Embrace the forms of spirituality that make you feel peaceful and hopeful; they are what will allow your body to best heal.

References

Pew Research Religion and Public Life Project, *Religion and the Unaffiliated,* October 9, 2012. www.pewforum.org/2012/10/09/nones-on-the-rise-religion/, accessed October 12, 2014.

H. G. Koenig, "Religion, Spirituality, and Health: The Research and Clinical Implications," *ISRN Psychiatry* 2012 (December 16, 2012), doi:10.5402/2012/278730.

J. R. Peteet and M. J. Balboni, "Spirituality and Religion in Oncology," *CA: A Cancer Journal for Clinicians* 63, no. 4 (July–August 2013): 280–89.

H. G. Koenig and H. J. Cohen, *The Link between Religion and Health: Psychoneuroimmunology and the Faith Factor* (Oxford: Oxford University Press, 2002), pp. 11, 25.

J. Moon, *How to Pray without Being Religious* (London: HarperCollins, 2005), p. 11.

S. L. Carter, "The Power of Prayer, Denied," *New York Times*, January 31, 1996, p. A17.

"Faith Healers Sentenced in Daughter's Death," *New York Times*, June 11, 1997, p. A23.

W. Nolen, *Healing: A Doctor in Search of a Miracle* (New York: Random House, 1974).

J. Randi, *The Faith Healers* (Amherst, NY: Prometheus Books, 1989), pp. 139–42.

T. J. Connerty and V. Knott, "Promoting Positive Change in the Face of Adversity: Experiences of Cancer and Post-traumatic Growth," *European Journal of Cancer Care* (England) 22, no. 3 (May 2013): 334–44.

P. A. Sealy, "Integrating Job, Jesus' Passion, and Buddhist Metta to Bring Meaning to the Suffering and Recovery from Breast Cancer," *Journal of Religion and Health* 52, no. 4 (December 2013): 1162, 1165–67.

J. K. Silver, *What Helped Get Me Through: Cancer Survivors Share Wisdom and Hope* (Atlanta, GA: American Cancer Society, 2009), pp. 177–202.

J. Groopman, "God at the Bedside," *New England Journal of Medicine* 350 (2004): 1176–78.

L. Dossey, *Prayer Is Good Medicine* (New York: HarperCollins, 1996), pp. 81–83.

J. Offner, "Pow-Wowing: The Pennsylvania Dutch Way to Heal," *Journal of Holistic Nursing* 16 (1998): 483.

M. Thibodeaux, *God, I Have Issues: 50 Ways to Pray No Matter How You Feel* (Cincinnati, OH: St. Anthony Messenger Press, 2005), p. 62.

L. Dossey, *Healing Beyond the Body* (Boston: Shambhala, 2001), p. 222.

H. Benson, *The Relaxation Response* (New York: HarperCollins, 2000), pp. 12–13.

L. S. Das, *Letting Go of the Person You Used to Be* (New York: Broadway Books, 2003), p. 18.

L. Eib, *When God and Cancer Meet* (Wheaton, IL: Tyndale House, 2002), pp. 170, 173, 177.

CHAPTER 13

LOVE AND

BE LOVED

A strong support network of family and friends is consistently cited as one of the most important factors in maintaining a good quality of life. Increasingly, we are recognizing the part that friendship, love, and support play in maintaining good health and in healing after an illness. People who lack intimate relationships and strong friendships, regardless of their physical health, consistently report higher rates of depression and dissatisfaction with their lives. Renowned heart specialist Dr. Dean Ornish, writing of the healing power of love and intimacy in his bestseller *Love and Survival*, says, "If a new drug had the same impact, virtually every doctor in the country would be recommending it for their patients. It would be malpractice not to prescribe it." Dr. Ornish was referring to the many studies that clearly show a relationship between overall health—including immune system function—and social relationships.

It is also possible that our connections with others may influence our ability to survive cancer. For example, a study that was presented by Dr. Karen Weihs at a meeting of the American Psychosomatic Society and reported in *USA Today* followed women with Stage II breast cancer for seven years. Dr. Weihs found that the women who had a larger support network had a significantly improved survival rate. Although this study is not conclusive, it suggests (as some other studies have) that survival may be influenced by support from family, friends, support groups, and other human connections. A subsequent *Cochrane*

Database Systematic Review looked at ten randomized control trials that were performed in women with metastatic (advanced) breast cancer. Seven of the studies included involved group therapy. In this review, the researchers concluded that psychological interventions appeared to be effective in improving survival at twelve months but not at longer-term follow-up—meaning that women who received psychosocial support were more likely to be alive at the one year mark. They noted that the results should be interpreted with caution since more research in this area is needed.

Yet, cancer can wreak havoc with relationships. Cancer can, and often does, strip people of what they hold dear—their cherished relationships with partners, children, siblings, extended family members, and friends. Jennie Nash was diagnosed with breast cancer at age 35. After her recovery, she wrote about how "cancer gives people a great opportunity to rise to the occasion—to be present, to be understanding, to tell you all the things they never said before. . . . [T]he lesson is to let them." Nash was fortunate enough to have a close contingent of family and friends watch over her as she went through several complicated surgical procedures including a mastectomy and breast reconstruction. During this time of intense stress, however, Nash's husband and her mother battled bitterly. Nash recounts in her memoir, *The Victoria's Secret Catalog Never Stops Coming*, that, despite a previously good relationship, "now, as I lay in a bed in a critical care unit of a hospital, bleeding into my belly, their fury at each other grew so strong they couldn't even sleep in the same house."

Joyce Wadler, another woman who faced breast cancer and wrote about it (in *My Breast*), tells of her oncologist's response when she tearfully told her of how she had broken up with her boyfriend. Her doctor sympathized, "You know, this happens with a lot of women after they have a diagnosis of cancer. . . . They look at their relationships; they reassess them. A lot of people break up. And then, on top of that, you have the stress of the disease, making everything worse."

When I was diagnosed with cancer, my life came to a screeching halt. I instantly realized that I would be devoting—at a minimum—the next year of my life to trying to recover from this illness. Under normal circumstances, I enjoy meeting new people and sharing my life with others. During my treatment and recovery, however, my life was not about making new friends, but rather it focused on simply making it through each day. I didn't have the energy to socialize with anyone except my closest friends and loved ones. I had treated many people with serious medical conditions, and I had heard them tell how their social world shriveled. But still, when I was diagnosed with cancer myself, I was surprised to see just how much my world consisted of people whose lives I had touched *before* I was sick. Joni Rodgers, a young woman diagnosed with non-Hodgkin's lymphoma, sums it up this way in *Bald in the Land of Big Hair*: "Hi, I'm Joni, and I'm a sucking black hole of emotional need right now. My hobbies are taking drugs, napping, and calling people I hardly know for emergency child-care. Wanna be my friend?"

As Rodgers suggests, people with cancer tend to have difficulty reaching out to others. There may be many individual reasons for their lack of sociability; let's begin trying to put the matter into perspective by taking a look at how cancer and other diseases were viewed in the past. Historically, almost every serious illness was associated with shame and the belief that the person suffering somehow deserved to bear this cross. The "blame-the-victim" mentality persisted for thousands of years and was present in many different religious and cultural belief systems. In *A Darker Ribbon*, Ellen Leopold examines the political and social history of breast cancer: "The belief in disease as a divine punishment for sin (or for any form of moral 'uncleanliness') opened the door to extreme forms of human punishment. . . . Leprosy, whose disfiguring symptoms could not easily be hidden away, was considered to be retribution for the sin of lust. Lepers were literally banished from society."

It is not surprising, then, that through the centuries many (if not all) serious illnesses have caused people to withdraw from their families and loved ones. People diagnosed with cancer have a long tradition of hiding their symptoms. You may be thinking that this reaction is passé and that cancer, once a taboo subject, has actually become in some circles a badge of honor. Unfortunately, remnants of shame still affect some of us who are seriously ill. For example, one of my patients is a disabled young man who lived in poverty in Vietnam until he was a teenager. He told me that, while he was in Vietnam, those around him believed he had done something terrible to deserve his fate. They considered his presence "bad luck," and he was not allowed to attend school or go to birthday parties, weddings, or funerals. He had never been to a single social event until he came to the United States.

Of course, people who have lived in the United States their entire lives also experience abandonment by loved ones. There are plenty of cancer survivors who have stories of loved ones who were not able to accept their illness and the complications that it entailed and literally walked out on their sick partner, friend, or colleague. When I was initially diagnosed, I talked to a colleague's wife who had been through breast cancer a decade earlier. She told me that her dearest friend had stopped contacting her during her illness and that they never regained their intimate friendship. Her friend later told her, "I just couldn't handle it."

Fortunately, I didn't have to face this kind of rejection. My loved ones rallied to help and support me. The hard part for me wasn't finding people willing to help but rather *allowing* them to do so. I wanted to cook for my children and take them to their after-school activities. I wanted to take care of my patients, too. But I couldn't do everything that I did before I was diagnosed. Indeed, I couldn't manage to do most of what I usually did. Instead, I had to find a graceful way of accepting help and letting those who loved me show me how much they cared. It wasn't easy.

Out of necessity, however, I did accept help. And, in doing so, I started to think that whenever people offered me help it was because they knew about my illness and were trying to ease the burden. I realized that my perspective needed to be adjusted when I wrongly assumed that a lovely woman, a new friend of mine, was being nice to me because she had heard I was ill. I later realized that she had no idea I had cancer and was simply a terrific person who likes to help others.

One of my patients, a man who has faced serious health problems, sent me a letter in which he wrote about former president Jimmy Carter's struggle to share his "private recesses" with other people. His letter included these comments:

I just finished reading Jimmy Carter's latest book, *Sharing Good Times*, about the things in life that matter most, "the simple, relaxed days and nights . . . enjoyed with family and friends through the years and across generations." If you haven't read it I'd recommend that you do.

In his book, President Carter shares how he has had to work at including others in his daily activities, learning to "stretch mind and heart and to combine work and pleasure." His book has inspired me as I, too, am learning to live life at a different pace, discovering the joy of sharing time and activities with my family and friends.

I relate closely to President Carter's own experience, summed up in his book's Introduction: "the main lesson I have struggled to learn is that the experiences (of life) are more deep and lasting sources of pleasure when they are shared with others. It has not been easy for me to accept this fact. Perhaps like most other people, I have had to overcome a self-centered inclination to live on my own terms, sometimes obsessed with intense ambition, bringing others into the private recesses of my life only reluctantly. I've come to realize that even my loved ones and I could enjoy the same event without really sharing the essence of it, and that it takes a lot of effort to sense and accommodate the desires of others in a generous way. This lifetime of learning has paid rich dividends for me and for those with whom I have learned to really share."

I appreciate Jimmy Carter's words and recognize that I am on a similar journey, learning to include others in my work and play.

Unfortunately, my patient will have the opportunity to put this lesson into practice, as his wife was diagnosed with colon cancer shortly after he wrote this letter. Thankfully, she is expected to do well.

COUPLES AND INTIMACY

Couples often experience dramatic changes in their relationships following a serious illness in one partner, because of the intensity of their feelings for each other and the amount of time they spend together. Studies have yielded conflicting results about whether a cancer diagnosis leads to a higher divorce rate among married couples, but any life-threatening illness puts an enormous strain on both people in a close relationship.

There are many reasons that emotional and physical intimacy may be affected by cancer and its treatment. For example, cancer can lead to embarrassment about an altered body image due to loss of a body part (a breast, a testicle, or an extremity) or disfigurement (as in head and neck cancers) or weight gain or loss; changing roles of the partners, so that one becomes more of a caretaker; or depression or other emotional problems in either partner. One of my colleagues, Jennifer Potter, wrote an essay coauthored by her wife, who was diagnosed with acute myelogenous leukemia. The two women, who are intensely devoted to each other, discussed how they faced some of these difficult issues. They recalled one conversation in which Dr. Potter's wife said, "I don't look like me anymore—I look grotesque. How can you love me?"

Survivors of cancers with a hormonal component, such as endometrial, ovarian, breast, and prostate cancer, may experience decreased libido due to changes in hormone levels. Men with testicular or prostate cancer may find it difficult to achieve or maintain an erection. Pain can be a factor both in a person's physical ability to be intimate and in the emotional willingness to seek out intimacy. I discussed the impact of pain on couples' intimacy in my book *Chronic Pain and the Family*:

> Chronic pain has a marked effect on people's ability to remain intimate and sexually active. This is an issue for both the person in pain and the healthy partners. Although intimacy means different things to everyone, it goes far beyond sexual intercourse. Intimacy is the way that couples relate to each other—both physically and emotionally. Sexuality may involve special looks that couples give each other, verbal communication, caresses, and finally the sex act itself. . . . A majority of people with chronic pain report reduced sexual interest and satisfaction. In some studies, more than 80 percent of patients and their spouses report significant reduction in or elimination of sexual activity.

Intimacy can be affected by the specific cancer type, the stage of the illness, treatment (altered hormone levels) and treatment side effects (such as pain and fatigue), and medications used to lessen side effects of the treatment (see Tables 13.1 and 13.2). It may also be affected by emotional responses such as anxiety and depression. Finally, any preexisting problems in the relationship are often exacerbated.

Table 13.1. Cancer-Related Intimacy Factors

Effects of the Disease

Weight loss, muscle loss

Anemia

Anxiety or depression

Bowel or bladder incontinence

Neurological impairments (for example, injury to the brain or to nerves elsewhere in the body)

Abdominal, pelvic, or chest pain or swelling

Loss of sensation

Effects of Treatment

Fatigue

Nausea

Pain

Hair loss

Disfigurement or loss of body parts

Decreased libido (sexual interest)

Erectile dysfunction

Decreased vaginal lubrication

Decreased or absent ability to achieve orgasm

Weight gain or loss

Effects of Medications Used to Ease the Side Effects of Treatment

Decreased libido

Difficulty obtaining or maintaining an erection

Decreased ability to achieve orgasm

Fatigue

Decreased vaginal lubrication

Weight gain or loss

For most cancer survivors, particularly those who are finished with cancer treatments and are in the recovery phase, there are no medical reasons to avoid physical intimacy. Exceptions might include the weeks following surgery or when a partner's immune system is unstable enough that no close contact of any kind is safe. There may also be a period during treatment when the person is too sick to be physically intimate. However, some people will want to maintain physical intimacy throughout their course of treatment and may find it very reassuring to

Table 13.2. Some Classes of Drugs That May Affect Sexual Function	
Antianxiety medications	Diuretics
Antidepressants	Hormonal medications
Antihistamines	Illicit street drugs
Antinausea medications	Muscle relaxants
Blood pressure medications	Pain medications
Cardiac medications	Sleep medications
Chemotherapeutic agents	

resume as soon as possible after surgery or continue while other therapies are ongoing.

Also keep in mind that even if you anticipate infertility as a consequence of your cancer treatment, you should use contraception if you are not interested in conceiving a child (unless, of course, you are certain that one partner is infertile). Infertility may not always result when it is expected, so you should be diligent about avoiding an unwanted pregnancy.

If you and your loved one are struggling with emotional or physical intimacy, or both, there are a number of ways you can improve the situation. Of course, if your problems are long-standing and predate the cancer diagnosis, the underlying issues will need to be addressed. For couples who had a stable and loving relationship prior to cancer, however, the following section may help.

IMPROVING INTIMACY

It is likely that, over the past weeks and months, your conversations with your partner—far more of them than previously—have been about health-related issues. Both the content and the way in which conversations flow may be altered: one person may be trying to protect the other, or one person (or both) may feel sad, worried, or depressed. Reconnecting emotionally with your partner is about both what you say and what you do. Table 13.3 lists some suggestions for improving emotional intimacy. Physical intimacy, whether it involves sexual intercourse or not, is also an important part of most couples' relationships. See Table 13.4 for some practical suggestions for enhancing physical intimacy.

Table 13.3. Enhancing Emotional Intimacy

Set aside time to have a conversation about issues you have been avoiding or issues that are emotionally charged. During this "date" be encouraging to your partner and listen to him or her at least as much as you talk. Sharing your feelings is a great way to build emotional intimacy.

Do something together that doesn't involve a lot of verbal communication. Go to a movie or a concert.

Take time to enjoy nature together. Have a picnic, take an outdoor hike, or go for a walk or a bike ride.

Join something together, such as a cooking or foreign language class.

Go out for a nonalcoholic drink at your favorite coffee shop.

Plan a romantic dinner at a local restaurant.

Read to each other.

Do a crossword puzzle together or play a board game.

Table 13.4. Enhancing Physical Intimacy

Great sex is a whole-body experience—or more precisely, a body, mind, and soul experience.

Remember that your most important sexual organ is between the ears. Sexiness is at first mental, then it goes somewhere else.

Both partners need to be aroused to have a good experience. Play to your partner's dominant sense (sight, sound, or touch) to heighten his or her arousal.

Make it easier to get an erection by using positions in lovemaking that take advantage of gravity, thus helping blood flow into the penis.

If you have partial erections, try partial penetration.

Take turns pleasing each other. Loving means giving and receiving.

Sensual touching is extremely arousing for most couples. Use touching to learn about each other's touch points for arousal. Touch each other for the sheer pleasure of it.

Both partners can have orgasms without intercourse.

Visualization and fantasy can enhance your sex life.

Creative ideas and novelty are two keys to creating and maintaining self-renewal relationships.

Source: Excerpt from Ralph and Barbara Alterowitz. *Intimacy with Impotence: The Couple's Guide to Better Sex after Prostate Disease* (Cambridge, MA: Perseus, 2004), p. 57.

Intimacy is obviously a complicated and emotionally charged subject. If it is an issue for you, then talk to your doctor about what is troubling you. Your doctor has almost certainly had many discussions with patients about intimacy and will likely be able to offer some insight and helpful advice. For suggestions about the kinds of questions you might want to broach with your doctor, see Table 13.5.

You may also want to consider other professional help with intimacy issues. Cancer centers often offer sexual rehabilitation services such as an evaluation of the physical problems that might contribute to dif-

---

Table 13.5. Questions about Intimacy and Infertility to Ask Your Doctor

For Women
Will cancer treatment leave me with a temporary or permanent loss of sensation? If so, what can I expect?
Will I experience painful intercourse (due to reduced vaginal lubrication or changes in the genital tissue)? If so, what can I do about the changes?
Will I undergo premature menopause? If so, how can I treat the symptoms?

For Men
Will I have less feeling in my genitals? If so, how will it affect me?
Will I be left impotent or have difficulty maintaining an erection or ejaculating? If so, what can I do about the situation?

For Men and Women of Childbearing Age
How will my cancer or the treatment affect my fertility?
Can I freeze my sperm or eggs?
What are my options for having children after treatment?

For Everyone
When can I safely resume sexual activity?
Will I experience less sexual desire (decreased libido)?
Will I experience less physical pleasure with intimacy and sexual intercourse?
Are there any special precautions that I should take?
Will any of the medications (or other treatments) I am currently taking affect me emotionally or physically with regard to intimacy?
Are my issues with intimacy going to be permanent?
Can you offer me suggestions (about creams, medications, devices, etc.) on how to improve my ability to be physically intimate?
Can you refer me to a professional who specializes in the type of intimacy issues that I am dealing with?

---

ficulty with sexual intercourse and counseling for those who are dealing with emotional issues that can impact intimacy. Sexual dysfunction clinics may be conducted by your local hospital or a private group in your area. These clinics typically offer the same types of services as a cancer center does and can include health professionals such as gynecologists, urologists, endocrinologists, psychiatrists, psychologists, and clinical social workers. Sex therapy, another option, usually involves working as a couple with a mental health professional for a specific period (usually around ten to twenty visits). The goal of sex therapy is to treat issues specifically related to intimacy. Underlying marital problems are better addressed in traditional couples therapy. For more information on resources, see the appendix.

Regardless of where you are in terms of your treatment, improving intimacy with your partner is an important goal. Physical intimacy is a significant part of most adult couples' relationships, despite age and illness. But cancer can and does get in the way. As psychologist Leslie Schover writes in *Sexuality and Infertility after Cancer*, "Sex and cancer are two words that do not seem to belong in the same sentence. We think of sexuality as a force for joy and new life, whereas cancer is a death force. Increasingly, however, men and women survive their cancers. . . . Being able to enjoy sex is one important battle in winning the war against cancer."

Note also the part that nonsexual physical intimacy can play. Joyce and Barry Vissell (a nurse and a psychiatrist, respectively) write in *The Heart's Wisdom: A Practical Guide to Growing through Love*, "Snuggling, hugging, and touching each other (especially in a non-sexual way) is an essential ingredient for every relationship. . . . Such a simple act can carry much power to sustain and heal our relationships far beyond what the mind thinks possible."

FERTILITY

The ability to conceive a child is an issue with many different types of cancer, may affect both men and women, and can result from both adult and childhood cancers and treatments. Infertility can also be seen as a tragic consequence (a "double whammy") of surviving a life-threatening disease. For some people infertility is a terrific loss and may bring about intense feelings of sadness, shame, worry, and anger. Just the possibility of future infertility can interfere with relationships. As one of my patients who had Hodgkin's lymphoma as a child says, "At what point do you tell someone you are dating that you might not be able to have children?" The inability to have the family you always dreamed of can be a terrible blow. Coupled with an uncertain future and your own brush with mortality, it can be genuinely devastating.

Infertility may come as a surprise or may be an expected outcome of the cancer treatment. It may also be temporary, for example, when a young woman with breast cancer goes into menopause during chemotherapy treatment and then several weeks or months after the end of treatment resumes ovulation and menstruation. Sometimes a couple can plan ahead and "bank" frozen sperm or eggs. This procedure is not always helpful, though: for example, a woman with uterine cancer who has her uterus removed still won't be able to carry a child—though engaging a surrogate mother might be an option. The good news is that there is an increasing emphasis in survivorship care on preserving fertility, and new research is helping to pave the way for cancer survivors. Dr. Brian Foley, my colleague quoted in chapter 2 (writing about healing, he said he would "cultivate the garden of me" and focus "not exclusively on the weeds [tumor], but on nourishing and supporting the garden"), describes receiving his diagnosis of oral cancer through a fax that his doctor sent to his home and how his thoughts immediately focused on his future ability to raise children: "I read aloud, 'squamous cell carcinoma tumor present on all margins.' . . . I was shocked. No denial. No disbelief. I felt only anger. Some say there is a reason for everything. That was not an acceptable explanation for me. What was the reason for this? Why did Linda [his wife] have to get this news? She deserved better. Would we ever have our own children? Would I make my young wife a single mother and widow?"

Regardless of whether you already have children, the loss of the ability to have more may be a severe blow. A childhood friend of mine had a hysterectomy to treat cervical cancer. She has five children, but she had planned on having a very large family. Another woman I know had a similar procedure for cervical cancer, has one child and also had intended to expand her family in the future. Each woman talked to me about how devastated she was to have her uterus removed. The number of children they each already had didn't impact their feeling of loss.

If you are concerned about childbearing issues, talk to your doctor and seek out specialists in the area of reproductive medicine. This field is rapidly changing, so there may be options for you that you didn't realize existed. The more information you have, the better you will be able to make a decision that is right for you and your family.

What to Tell Children about Cancer

Cancer is a family disease. There is no way to keep children, whatever their ages, from being affected by their parent's cancer. Although this section is written from the perspective of a parent, much of the information may be applicable to readers who are grandparents, aunts, uncles or have other close relationships with children. Wendy Schlessel Harpham, a physician, was a young mother when she was diagnosed with non-Hodgkin's lymphoma. In her book *When a Parent Has Cancer*, she reminds us that "the greatest gift you can give your children is not protection from change, loss, pain, or stress, but the confidence and tools to cope and grow with all that life has to offer them." Here are a few guidelines for helping your children through this ordeal:

Tell them the name of your disease and use the word cancer. All children should be given the name of any serious illness. For cancer, it is best to use this word, since they'll almost certainly hear it elsewhere. I vividly recall a relaxing walk I was taking with my then 7-year-old daughter. We bumped into a woman I knew but hadn't seen in a while. With my daughter standing wide-eyed by my side, she exclaimed, "I heard you had *cancer*. How *awful!* You must be so *scared!*" There was no way to protect my daughter from this person, and I was glad I had told her ahead of time that we would hear things like this. Because she heard that I had cancer from me first, in a safe context, the impact of this well-meaning woman's remarks was reduced.

Remember, you are your children's best source of information. Also keep in mind that all children have a real sense of when someone is being honest with them. Always tell them the truth. Don't keep a cancer diagnosis a secret. You don't have to tell them everything at once, as they may not have the attention span to listen to all of the details. But make sure that whatever you tell them is the truth. Dr. Harpham notes, "When the facts are couched in love and hopefulness, you can guide your children toward a life-enhancing perception of reality. In the end, that's what parenting is all about."

If you are in the process of raising your children, you have every right to be worried about them. Hester Hill Schnipper, an oncology social worker and breast cancer survivor, offers parents this reassurance, however, in her book *After Breast Cancer*:

> It is very likely that your children will have adjusted quickly and managed reasonably well during your months of treatment. I and colleagues in my hospital's Department of Psychiatry worked on a longitudinal study of the reactions of children to a mother's breast cancer, and we have found, over and over, that children who are given age-appropriate information and whose routines remain consistent do very well. Indeed, their mothers say that it sometimes seems as if the children actually forget about the cancer and so are startled when they catch a glimpse of a bald head or are told of a doctor's appointment. They do not really forget, of course, nor are they in denial. It is simply that their healthy defenses are working well, protecting them as they go about their daily business of growing up.

One of my colleagues, Dr. Paula Rauch, is a child psychiatrist who directs the cancer center parenting program at Massachusetts General Hospital in Boston. In her book, *Raising an Emotionally Healthy Child When a Parent Is Sick*, she discusses the importance of getting children back to some kind of routine—even if it's different from their old routine, being able to count on a schedule provides some stability. She also says that good parenting, whether you are sick or healthy, is basically the same. However, you should have contingency plans that will help your children and the rest of your family deal with uncertainty when you are sick. I asked her what she most wanted parents to know about helping their children. She replied:

> I encourage parents to focus on three arenas of a child's life: the child's schedule, family time, and communication. Have a predictable daily and weekly routine, because this makes the world feel safer to a child. Turn off

the phone during meals, and protect family time from too many visitors or phone conversations about a parent's health status. Be honest and simple about illness explanations and encourage children to ask their own questions. Welcome all questions warmly and try to tease out the real question a child has before launching into an answer that may not address the real concern or confusion. When you focus on these three arenas, often the parent's illness recedes into the background and the focus turns to the child's healthy development.

Tell them about cancer using words they understand. Dr. Rauch also remarked that children need honest and up-to-date information about their parent's diagnosis: "A common error of kindness happens when parents imagine that not talking about their cancer protects their child from worry. Instead the child is likely to overhear information about the parent's illness and be left thinking either the parent does not care enough about the child to speak to him directly or that the news is too hard to discuss. In each of these scenarios, the child is left to worry alone and is more likely to assume confused or inaccurate information."

Specifically, children need to know that cancer is not contagious and that it is not their fault that you have the disease. These two points often get missed, and children will frequently answer these questions for themselves—possibly coming up with erroneous conclusions. Give details about what you expect to happen now and in the future. You don't have to explain all of this at once, but it is advisable to tell them right away that you are getting help from your doctor and that although you may have to live with cancer for a long time, or possibly forever, you are trying new treatments that you hope will help. If there are noticeable side effects, explain them. Discuss your prognosis, or they'll come to their own conclusions. Children can imagine all kinds of scenarios including that they'll be given up for adoption—regardless of your prognosis. So, if you are hopeful that you'll live a long life, tell them that. The book *Cancer in the Family*, by the American Cancer Society, includes some excellent suggestions on how to respond to the question "Are you going to die?" (see Table 13.6). If your children don't ask this question, it is usually worthwhile to bring it up for discussion.

Explain how cancer affects your moods and your ability to participate

Table 13.6. Answering a Child's Question: "Are You Going to Die?"

Sometimes people do die from cancer. I'm not expecting that to happen because the doctors have told me they have very good treatments these days.

Many people are cured of cancer these days; that's why I'm getting treatment.

The doctors have told me that my chances of being cured are very good. I think we should believe them until they tell us otherwise. I'll let you know if that changes.

There is no way to know right now what's going to happen until I get some treatment. I think we should feel positive about things for now, and hopefully we will feel even better in the future.

Years ago, people often died from cancer because treatments weren't as good. Now there are a lot more choices of treatment, and the outlook for many cancers is much more hopeful.

They don't know a lot about the kind of cancer I have. But I'm certainly going to give it my best.

My cancer is a tough one to treat, but I'm going to work hard at getting better. We just don't know what is going to happen. The most important thing is that we stick together as a family and let each other know what's going on with all of us. If you can't stop worrying, I want you to tell me because there are things we can do to feel better.

I don't think I'm going to die. None of us knows for sure. But I'm going to do everything I can to make sure that doesn't happen.

Source: Sue P. Heiney, Joan F. Herman, Katherine V. Bruss, and Joy L. Fincannon, *Cancer in the Family* (Atlanta, GA: American Cancer Society, 2001), p. 14.

in your children's lives. Children need to know what to expect from their parents. Tell your children what you can and can't do—especially as it pertains to family routines and special occasions. Let them know that your love and devotion to them are unchanged despite the fact that you must spend time going to the doctor or dealing in other ways with your illness. Explain that your moods are not their fault and that you are working to become emotionally stable. Emphasize that you are still their parent, despite your condition.

The amount of detail your children will need to know will vary depending on their age, maturity, and ability to understand the explanation. See the following sections for more about how they might react according to their age. In the beginning, just tell them what you think they can grasp. Then bring the subject up again every few weeks or when some significant change is scheduled (for example, surgery or some other procedure). This way, you keep the lines of communication open and give your children the opportunity to ask additional questions. Although I expected new things to come up with all of my children over time, I was still a little surprised when it took two years for my youngest child to tell me, "I thought you were going to die." When I was diagnosed, she was 3 years old. Two years later, she was far more sophisticated and articulate. If you are concerned about your children's reactions, see subsequent sections of this chapter for warning signs that they may need professional help.

Undeniably it can be difficult to help your children when you are in the midst of a serious illness. One of the best pieces of advice I ever heard a psychologist give a parent was that *your children will do as well as you do*. This advice pertains to emotional, rather than physical, health. Children generally take their cues from their parents. If you are positive, hopeful, honest, and communicative, your children will likely be resilient and weather your cancer fairly well. Listen to your children. Stay in tune with what is happening to them at home and at school. Finally, seek professional help if you feel that your child's problems are beyond the scope of what is normal and what you are able to address at home.

The Very Young Child

For toddlers and preschool-age children, begin with just the essential details. You can use dolls or stuffed animals to help them understand your illness. This "play technique" has been found to be effective with young children. You may also use words that they understand, such as *boo-boo*, rather than more technical terms.

Because children at this age are involved in "magical thinking" (they often believe that just by thinking something they can make it happen), it is important to tell them that they didn't do anything to cause Mommy or Daddy to be sick. That they are not responsible in any way for your illness if they get mad at you or don't do what they are asked to do. Also, explain that they are not in danger and that they will not "catch" cancer.

Choose a calm time when your child isn't tired or hungry and choose a setting without too many distractions. You may not be able to explain all that you have in mind in one sitting. That is fine—it is best to not go beyond your child's attention span. If you need to stop because your toddler's attention has wandered or your preschooler is squirming, then bring up the subject at another time when you think she or he is ready to hear more. Remember that children in this age group may not fully comprehend or recall even the simplest details, so be prepared to repeat yourself several times. You can also anticipate that whatever you tell your child will probably be repeated to others—possibly inaccurately.

The Older Child

School-age children will be able to understand more about what is happening. Once again, start with basic information about the name of your condition and what you expect to happen now and in the future. Simple diagrams and explanations from books and websites can help. Again, review that your cancer is not your child's fault and that he or she can't catch it from you. Once you have provided this information, give some details about what is happening in your family. Who is going to take care of this child's needs? Who will drive him or her to school, help with homework, make the meals, and so forth? Although it would be ideal to keep things the same as before your illness, often routines will change. *Let your school-age child know how things are going to change and how he or she will be affected.*

If you have ongoing medical treatment, you may want to take your child with you to a doctor's or other appointment, giving her or him further opportunities to ask questions and learn about what is going on. School-age children should be told something about their parent's prognosis. If you and your doctor believe that your symptoms will improve with treatment, then share that with your child; but, once again, be honest.

The Adolescent Child

Adolescents have a much greater understanding of medical problems, but their information may not be accurate—especially if it was gleaned from the media or from friends. It is essential that you give accurate information to your child. Because adolescence is a time of crucial identity formation and establishing independence, illness in a parent can be confusing to a teen—your child may feel torn between newfound autonomy and the need to stay close to home during a crisis. Adolescents are ready for very detailed explanations. All of their questions should be answered as honestly and completely as possible. If the illness is causing tension in the family, bring this up. Give your adolescent child the most realistic explanation possible, and state clearly what is expected of him or her.

It is also a good idea to make sure that adolescents have someone outside the immediate family circle to confide in—someone to whom they can express normal emotions that they might feel selfish, disloyal, or guilty about voicing within the family. Moreover, because adolescence is usually a time of great emotional turmoil even without having a parent who is seriously ill, children in this age group should be carefully watched to see whether they might need help from a professional counselor.

HOW TO TELL WHETHER YOUR CHILD NEEDS HELP

Various warning signs may indicate that your child needs professional help in dealing with her or his emotions and with your illness. Of course, your family members, especially children, must have the medical and psychological attention they need as they struggle with the day-to-day issues that arise when a parent has cancer. Treatment should focus on the whole family and is generally more successful for everyone when this is the case. Parents who see their children become casualties of their illness may feel guilty or depressed and have a harder time with their physical recovery than parents who take a proactive role in promoting good mental health and coping skills for their children.

Mood Changes

As your family struggles with issues surrounding cancer, there will be times when family members feel glum or worried. In children, the time to worry is when these moods *become persistent or are present more than they have been in the past*. All of us, including children, have a baseline mood level that fluctuates with events in our lives. When good things happen, we feel happier; when bad things happen, we are sad. In children, as in adults, the baseline mood level depends on their individual personalities. The warning sign to look for is a change in your child's prevailing mood. If you see such a change, then he or she needs some professional help.

New or Exaggerated Behaviors

You need to not only assess your child's mood but also look for new or exaggerated behaviors. For example, you should be concerned if your child who is usually outgoing becomes withdrawn or if your child begins to act out at home or at school. If your child is usually neat but begins to become obsessive about keeping his or her room clean, this change could be a warning sign. (The opposite change is just as significant.) If your child usually needs prompting to bathe but now completely disregards personal hygiene even with your reminders, you should consider whether she or he may need some counseling. You know your children better than anyone else, so you are the best judge of whether they have troubling new behaviors or exaggerated pre-existing habits that may need to be addressed by a professional.

Sleep Problems

In my home state of Massachusetts, there is a statewide test that all children must pass to graduate from high school. When children from a top-tier school were interviewed, I was struck by how much their teachers encouraged them to sleep. I had expected the children to report that they studied hard, but I was wrong. Instead, they said they were given little homework but were encouraged to sleep ten to twelve hours a night. The moral of this story is that the importance of sleep should never be underestimated.

Sleep problems take various forms depending on the age of the child. Most parents know when their children are having sleep problems— particularly when children have difficulty falling asleep or are getting up at night. Another sign of sleep disturbance is sleeping too much. If your child usually sleeps ten hours at night but suddenly can't get out of bed in the morning and wants to nap right after school, he or she may be clinically depressed. Your child needs professional help if you have tried to address sleep issues without success.

Increased or Decreased Appetite

Either an increase or a decrease in appetite may signal problems in children. Because the same changes may also be part of children's normal growth stages, the matter can be confusing. If you are worried, watch your child's mood for signals—be watchful not for a skipped meal here, a dinner of pizza and ice cream there, but for bigger patterns over weeks and months. Is your child gaining more weight than would be expected at this stage in development and given her or his level of activity? An increase in frequency and intensity of exercise, a fascination with the bathroom scale, and a penchant for looser clothing—especially if these behaviors appear suddenly—should be watched and set in a wider context of behavior and mood. Almost all kids (and adults for that matter) exhibit food preferences, but new eating quirks or obsession with the calories, as opposed to the nutrients, in food (for instance, counting the calories in breath mints, eating artificial sweetener from the packet as a snack) are highly suggestive and probably causes for concern.

In the absence of other worrying behaviors, children are the best regulators of what they eat, and parents are wise to carefully pick their battles when food is the issue (it is best to encourage your child to eat healthy food at meals but not to be overly critical of your child's eating habits). If you have a child who is overeating, then encourage her or him to exercise. Exercise has powerful benefits in promoting good health as well as improving one's mood. If your child is developing significant eating problems, get help sooner rather than later—particularly for teenagers, who are prone to serious eating disorders such as anorexia and bulimia (these can occur in preteen children as well).

Poor School Performance

One of the most critical messages to convey to your children regardless of their ages is the importance of doing well in school. Despite whatever is happening at home, they need to know that you expect them to continue to work hard at school. They need to know that you want

{ BEFORE AND AFTER CANCER TREATMENT }

them to focus on school and not on you. *They need your permission to keep academic work as a priority above and beyond the family's needs.* It is important to relieve them of any guilt they may have about spending time on their studies rather than on you or the family.

However, keeping school a priority is not always easy. I recall my son being very upset one night when my husband and I came home after a long day at the hospital. My son, usually very responsible, had forgotten to bring home a textbook he needed to study for a test the following day. It was late, and the school was locked up. We called one of his classmates, who readily agreed to lend him the book. But, by the time my husband picked it up, my son had little time to study for his test. Despite this episode and others that would not have occurred under normal circumstances, we concentrated on trying to keep school in first place for our children as much as possible.

Regardless of whatever else is going on, parents need to monitor home-work assignments and academic performance and to attend parent-teacher conferences just as they always have. Keep in mind that how well your children are performing at school is usually a good indicator of how they are doing otherwise. Although most children will act out at home during adolescence, they will likely weather their teens unscathed if they continue to display resilience and do acceptable work in school. But children who begin to perform poorly in school are at risk for significant problems in the future, and you should take such a change very seriously. Encouraging your children to go in the right direction is one of the best things you can do for your own health, because it alleviates stress and gives you something positive to focus on.

THE POWER OF FRIENDSHIP

Friends can enrich your life and help you to heal. Maybe they can help you live longer. In a fascinating study of a group of elderly Australians researchers found that friends, not family, were the most importal factor in survival. This research is not conclusive and does not addre friendship in cancer survivors, but it is interesting to consider how on relationships with others might impact health and healing. One th that is clear is that people with strong social networks have an impro quality of life.

Variety in friends seems to be an important factor as well as having an extensive network of friends. It is hard for anyone to meet all of your needs, so it is good to have supportive friends who are different from each other. Perhaps you have a friend who offers you helpful practical suggestions about the issues you are facing and another friend who plans fun outings and a third friend who thoroughly enjoys the role of "service" and helps you with chores and errands. Good friends are special, and each one has unique qualities that can help you during this time of recovery.

Although it might seem impossible to make new friends during this difficult time, you may come across wonderful opportunities to welcome unexpected friendships. One of my dearest friends tells me that she has no desire to make new friends. She is a terrific friend herself and has quite a few strong relationships with other people. When I asked her why she didn't want to embark on new relationships, she told me she was "all set." My friend's actions are contrary to her statement that she is all set, however: she is quite receptive to establishing new relationships. I have watched her over the years and have seen her develop wonderful friendships with various people.

The opportunity to connect with new people may come at any time, no matter if you are feeling tired, withdrawn, or "all set." Try to be receptive to the unexpected chance to make a new friend. One woman told me that she met her best friend as a stranger in a drugstore. The stranger noticed that she was bald and inquired about her illness. Both women had been through similar experiences, and the stranger-now-friend, a long-term cancer survivor, was a source of great inspiration and encouragement to this woman.

During your recovery, when your time and energy are limited, aim to spend time with friends who are able to do what some have labeled the "three Vs":

1. *Venture* forth and talk about what is important to you—including your illness.
2. *Validate* your feelings and concerns.
3. *Volunteer* to help you and your family during this difficult time.

{ BEFORE AND AFTER CANCER TREATMENT }

In a book titled *You've Got a Friend*, which one of my friends gave me during the time that I was healing, I ran across a great quote by English novelist George Eliot, who summed up the benefits of friendship in this way: "Oh, the comfort, the inexpressible comfort of feeling safe with a person, having neither to weigh thoughts nor measure words but to pour them all out, just as it is, chaff and grain together, knowing that a faithful hand will take and sift them, keeping what is worth keeping, and then, with the breath of kindness, blow the rest away."

SUPPORT GROUPS

In a landmark study that initially created a lot of excitement in the cancer community, researchers at Stanford University School of Medicine published data demonstrating that the women they had studied with metastatic breast cancer lived longer if they participated in support groups. In order for research to be conclusive, the results need to be repeated in other studies. Unfortunately, subsequent studies looking at survival in cancer patients have not consistently shown the same remarkable results.

Many studies have indicated, however, that people who participate in support groups tend to feel less worried, anxious, and depressed. Support group members also report a better quality of life and may feel less tired and have more vigor. But support groups are not for everyone. For example, John is a young man with an early-stage kidney (renal) cancer that was found by accident on an imaging study when he was being worked up for something else entirely. Renal cancer is usually diagnosed in men older than John and often at a more advanced stage. When John and his wife were considering whether he should attend a cancer support group, they discussed the fact that he might not feel comfortable attending a support group where he would be the youngest person present. They also thought about the likelihood that he would meet people whose prognosis was not nearly as promising as his; hearing about their less favorable prospects could be unsettling. It is perfectly reasonable for people to choose not to attend a support group if for any reason they might not feel comfortable.

John is fortunate in that he has a devoted wife and a large network of extended family and friends. Because he already has this group of supporters, he opted out of joining a support group. But many people whose situation is similar to John's don't have the same connections. For those individuals, even if they have early-stage cancer with an overwhelmingly positive prognosis, talking to others in a support group environment may be very beneficial. For those who are well connected, a support group may be appealing because of the kinship among cancer survivors and because it may be easier to talk about some difficult issues with people who are not emotionally involved. The bottom line on support groups is that you should consider joining one if it appeals to you. If you aren't sure, you can try it out for a session or two and see if you feel comfortable.

Another option is to consider talking to or e-mailing someone who has already been through cancer and survived. In 1952 Terese Lasser, a grandmother who was healthy and vivacious, underwent what she thought would be a biopsy of a benign breast lump. When she awakened from surgery, it turned out to have been a mastectomy for breast cancer. This occurrence was typical at that time: a patient would sign a consent form allowing the doctor to do whatever was necessary based on the pathology of the lump at the time of surgery. Author Walter Ross reported Lasser's later comment: "Overwhelmed by anxieties so acute and so bewildering that I all but drowned in them, my mind surged with questions—some very practical but with no practical answers forthcoming, some rather foolish but nevertheless terribly serious to me, and some so highly personal I could not even bring myself to put them into words. How I ached to talk to another woman who had had the same experience and come through it, and so could counsel, and reassure, and understand! But no such woman was available." This experience propelled Lasser to start Reach for Recovery, which is now part of the American Cancer Society and involves peer-to-peer connections and counseling.

SOCIAL CAPITAL

Social capital can be very helpful when you are recovering from cancer. This concept refers to your social network, which goes beyond your family connections and friendships. In a landmark book that highlights significant changes in society's social connectedness during the 1990s that are still ongoing, Harvard professor Robert Putnam defines social capital in his book *Bowling Alone* as "connections among individuals— social networks and the norms of reciprocity and trustworthiness that arise from them." Social capital can be used in a positive way to help people connect and live well. Or it can be destructive (for instance, in a gang context). Putnam notes, "The Golden Rule [of social capital] is one formulation of generalized reciprocity." He gives the example of the T-shirt slogan used by a fire department in Oregon to publicize their annual fund-raising effort: "Come to our breakfast, we'll come to your fire."

Kathleen Brehony is a psychotherapist who summed up Putnam's work and added her own comments on social capital in her book *Living a Connected Life*:

> Loneliness is rampant and the majority of us are bowling alone. Bowling alone? Did you know that bowling is the most popular sport in America? In 1996, more than 91 million Americans bowled, 25 percent more than voted in the 1998 congressional elections. Bowlers outnumber joggers, skiers, golfers, and soccer players by more than two to one. . . . More Americans are bowling than ever before (an increase in 10 percent from 1980 to 1993). Surprisingly, though, league bowling has plummeted by more than 40 percent during this same time period. If this trend continues, league bowling will vanish in the first decade of this new century. . . . Something is missing from our lives when we realize that our web of belonging—our contacts, support, friendship, and activity—is very small; that, in fact, our human connections don't much extend beyond work and family.

Brehony is careful to make the distinction between *social* loneliness and *emotional* loneliness. Social loneliness occurs when you travel and are in a strange city or when you move to a new town and haven't yet established connections with others. Emotional loneliness is feeling isolated and rejected. This latter type of loneliness can be devastating for a person going through a serious illness who does not have people to share the struggle with. Emotional loneliness can lead to depression and other problems, such as low self-esteem and social alienation.

No matter where you are in the healing process, remember that connecting with loved ones and strengthening existing connections with friends, colleagues, and social networks can provide an enormous boost to your emotional and physical health. Will Jenks is a testament to how powerful love can be when facing adversity. Jenks was a midshipman assigned to the USS *Shannon*, which had just completed an eight-week voyage from Norfolk to Copenhagen, Lisbon, and Guantanamo Bay, Cuba, during the summer of 1951. He was looking forward to returning to Holy Cross College in Worcester, Massachusetts; but, instead of returning to school, he clung to life in an iron lung—his body ravaged by the polio virus. Jenks became a quadriplegic, and though he never resumed his studies at Holy Cross, he gave the keynote address to the graduating class of 1954. While the president of the college, Rev. John E. Brooks, turned the pages of his speech, Jenks told his classmates and their families, "I think it's likely I am not the most seriously wounded among us, only the most conspicuously bandaged. Sooner or later every one of us will be made to feel flawed, inadequate, powerless. . . . What I continue to learn daily is that there is only one way to put Humpty Dumpty together again: Let yourself be loved."

Jenks went on to become a successful computer programmer and a living legend at Holy Cross, where he served as his class secretary for more than twenty-five years. In 1979 the college granted him an honorary degree, and in 1988 an anonymous donor made a gift in his name, contributing $1 million to endow a professorship in the English department.

Jenks's ideas predated Dr. Dean Ornish's now-famous work on love and healing; however, both men have been instrumental in teaching people about the importance of love in recovery. Ornish notes, "In short, anything that promotes a sense of love and intimacy, connection and community is healing." There is the added benefit that by reaching out to others, you not only help yourself but also potentially improve their health. When Jenks was offered the honorary degree, he was ambivalent about accepting it; but he agreed, stating, "Fate left me poor, love made me rich. And that truth is worth proclaiming."

References

D. Ornish, *Love and Survival* (New York: HarperCollins, 1998), pp. 3, 14.

M. Elias, "Friends May Make Breast Cancer More Survivable," *USA Today*, March 7, 2001.

M. Mustafa, A. Carson-Stevens, D. Gillespie, and A. G. Edwards, "Psychological Interventions for Women with Metastatic Breast Cancer, *Cochrane Database Systematic Review* 6 (June 4, 2013): CD004253.

J. Nash, *The Victoria's Secret Catalog Never Stops Coming* (New York: Penguin, 2002), p. 67.

J. Wadler, *My Breast* (New York: Simon and Schuster, 1997), p. 136.

J. Rodgers, *Bald in the Land of Big Hair* (New York: HarperCollins, 2002), p. 61.

E. Leopold, *A Darker Ribbon* (Boston: Beacon Press, 1999), p. 25.

J. Carter, *Sharing Good Times* (New York: Simon and Schuster, 2004), pp. xi–xii.

J. Silver, *Chronic Pain and the Family* (Cambridge, MA: Harvard University Press, 2004), p. 35.

L. R. Schover, *Sexuality and Fertility after Cancer* (New York: Wiley, 1997), p. xi.

J. Vissell and B. Vissell, *The Heart's Wisdom: A Practical Guide to Growing through Love* (Berkeley, CA: Conari Press, 1999), pp. 160–61.

J. D. Kort, M. L. Eisenberg, L. S. Millheiser, and L. M. Westphal, "Fertility Issues in Cancer Survivorship," *CA: A Cancer Journal for Clinicians* 64, no. 2 March–April 2014): 118–34.

B. S. Foley, *News from SPOHNC* 13 (2004): 4.

W. S. Harpham, *When a Parent Has Cancer* (New York: HarperCollins, 1997), pp. 8, 13.

H. H. Schnipper, *After Breast Cancer: A Common-Sense Guide to Life after Treatment* (New York: Random House, 2003), pp. 178–79.

P. K. Rauch and A. C. Muriel, *Raising an Emotionally Health Child When a Parent Is Sick* (New York: McGraw-Hill, 2005).

L. C. Giles et al., "Effect of Social Networks on 10 Year Survival in Very Old Australians: The Australian Longitudinal Study of Aging," *Journal of Epidemiological Community Health* 59 (2005): 574–79.

D. Zadra, *You've Got a Friend: Thoughts to Celebrate the Joy of Friendship* (Seattle, WA: Compendium, 2004), p. 12.

D. Spiegel et al., "Group Support for Patients with Metastatic Cancer: A Randomized Outcome Study," *Archives of General Psychiatry* 38 (1981): 527–33.

W. S. Ross, *Crusade* (New York: Arbor House, 1987), p. 161.

R. Putnam, *Bowling Alone* (New York: Simon and Schuster, 2000), pp. 19, 21.

K. Brehony, *Living a Connected Life* (New York: Holt, 2003), pp. 56–57.

W. J. Kane, *Let Yourself Be Loved: The Life and Letters of Will Jenks* (Saint Paul, MN: Syren, 2004), pp. xiii–xiv.

CHAPTER 14

SURMOUNT

SETBACKS

Being diagnosed with cancer is a ticket to a dangerous, sometimes thrilling, and always precarious roller coaster ride. If you
are a survivor, you have almost certainly experienced some of
the emotional highs and lows that are characteristic of the cancer experience. With the initial diagnosis there is, of course, shock and fear. As
time passes, the fear lessens if there are viable treatment options, and
the shock abates. That is not to say that things go back to the way they
were before the diagnosis, but rather that our minds find ways to adjust
to the situation at hand.

Just before I sat down to write this chapter, a woman whom I know
casually stopped me in a public place and informed me that her husband had been told the day before that he had lymphoma. He was lying
in a hospital bed and believed that his life was over. Both this woman
and her husband know that I am a doctor, and they had seen me from
time to time when I was going through my own treatment. Although I
had never openly discussed my diagnosis with them, they knew that I
was a cancer survivor. She told me on this day, "He has given up hope
and is asking to talk to you. He saw what you went through and he
believes you might be able to help him."

Practically everyone who has received a cancer diagnosis has gone
through what this family was now struggling with—the initial phase of
horror, fright, and despair. During this time, one's life is in limbo, be-

cause the diagnosis and the staging still need to be established. Treatment options are uncertain and the prognosis unclear.

The prognosis for people with lymphoma can vary greatly—as it can for nearly all types of cancer. It is quite possible that this family will be given promising news: that they can expect the lymphoma to respond favorably to treatment. If they get good news, their spirits will soar. No matter what, though, there will inevitably be hard times ahead.

I am often asked to talk to people right around the time of diagnosis. Inevitably, I tell them to ask their doctors about prehabilitation. In this book, I define prehabilitation and explain how it may help you to physically and emotionally get ready for upcoming cancer treatments. If you've already started cancer treatments, you can still ask your doctor about rehabilitation. Both prehabilitation and rehabilitation will *empower* you and help you to feel physically and emotionally stronger.

SETBACKS

Recall that early in this book I mentioned that setbacks are a part of the healing process. As a rehabilitation doctor, I treat many patients with serious injuries and illnesses. Some of the people who come to see me are what we call "multitrauma" patients: for instance, they might have been in a car accident and have sustained several injuries. It can take months or sometimes years to heal, and the road is usually not smooth. I often see other people who have a single, relatively straightforward medical problem, such as tendinitis. Even if the issue at hand is not terribly serious, the road to recovery may still be a bit bumpy. Thus, I frequently find myself telling patients that no matter how serious (or benign) a person's medical problems are, the recovery process typically includes periods of progress and other periods when the person seems to get worse instead of better. The setbacks can be relatively minor, difficulties that time will resolve, or they can be larger problems that require an adjustment in the treatment plan.

Carolyn Kaelin, my colleague who wrote about her illness in *Living through Breast Cancer*, described a number of setbacks during her own diagnosis and treatment. In the summer of 2003, Dr. Kaelin was 42 years old and training for the 190-mile Pan-Mass Challenge bike ride, a fund-raiser for cancer. Approximately two weeks before the ride, she noticed "the tiniest, most subtle area of skin pulling inward on my right breast." Although she didn't feel a lump, she did have breast cancer. Dr. Kaelin opted for breast-conserving surgery and underwent an initial lumpectomy, hoping that all of the cancer cells would be removed. They weren't. She had a second lumpectomy. Still, there were cancer cells remaining. A third lumpectomy failed as well. Finally, left with no other viable options, she underwent a mastectomy followed by a breast reconstruction surgery. Five surgeries after her initial diagnosis, Dr. Kaelin could move forward with the rest of her treatment and her recovery from breast cancer. Were her first few surgeries and the news that they didn't work setbacks? Sure. Do they mean that she doesn't have a good prognosis? Not necessarily. Setbacks in cancer treatment and recovery may have nothing to do with the ultimate prognosis. Nevertheless, they certainly can be discouraging.

Another colleague, who I mentioned previously, Dr. Ken Cohn, is a longtime cancer survivor. In 1980 he discovered a 3 cm mass in his neck. After surgical exploration he was diagnosed with "diffuse undifferentiated lymphoma." The abrupt transition from doctor to patient was difficult for Ken for a variety of reasons. Two years after his diagnosis, he wrote an article for the medical journal the *Lancet* called "Chemotherapy from an Insider's Perspective." In it he described how his doctors had difficulty communicating with him. Cohn wrote, "They seemed apprehensive about talking down to a patient with medical knowledge. This fear led to incomplete explanations of procedures about to be performed and to the failure to explain what complications to expect." Later in the essay Cohn gives a more specific example of how the lack of understanding affected him:

I was expected to receive ten courses of chemotherapy—the number of treatments most often used in this protocol. I was advised that aggressive treatment was the only way to eradicate lymphoma and that no-one ever survived a recurrence. However, 3 days after completing the eighth course of chemotherapy, I became so debilitated that I could not quicken my pace across the street when the traffic light changed. Even walking up half a flight of stairs made me [out of breath]. . . . I was told that I would receive no further chemotherapy. . . . The news that my treatments were finished produced no elation. I felt that, much as I dislike chemotherapy, my lifeline had been taken away from me. I felt that I had "failed the protocol."

The end of acute cancer treatment is often a time of confusion and sometimes despair for survivors. Although astute oncology health professionals recognize the perils associated with this transition, family members, friends, and indeed some healthcare providers may wrongly assume that the end of treatment signals a high point. It may be a mountaintop for some patients, but for others, like Dr. Cohn, it is a valley. Ironically, it was a colleague who helped Dr. Cohn sort out what it meant to end his treatments early. Cohn explains, "Not until a colleague told me that I had received at least as much medicine as any patient reported in the literature with my stage of disease and that the 7-year survival was 100% . . . did I begin to feel more secure."

Sometimes setbacks are physical issues related to the illness, as was the case with Drs. Kaelin and Cohn. Other times, the setback may be more emotionally based. For example, in April 2005 there was media frenzy around the report that a drug called Herceptin improved survival rates among women with breast cancer who had HER-2 positive tumor markers. To make this undeniably important news appear yet more exciting, the media went overboard in emphasizing how poor the prognosis generally was for women who were HER-2 positive. As I read the newspaper and listened to the radio, I thought how encouraging this news was for women currently undergoing treatment and receiving Herceptin but how discouraging the news was for women who might have been eligible for Herceptin but didn't get it.

One particularly disturbing report was an article in the May 9, 2005, issue of *Newsweek* that noted that HER-2 positive tumors "grow with unusual speed and are more likely to recur after treatment" (which is true). The article also quoted a woman for whom no credentials or identifying information was given other than her name: "hearing you have HER-2 is like hearing a death sentence." To suggest that women with HER-2 positive tumors have a "death sentence" is terribly misleading and simply wrong. The prognosis for women with breast cancer is dependent on many factors, only one of which is whether they are

HER-2 positive. Other factors include (but are not limited to) the stage of the cancer, whether it is estrogen receptor positive or not, and what treatment they choose to undergo. To report this wonderful research in a way that was alarming and not completely accurate was irresponsible and undoubtedly caused many women to have unnecessary emotional setbacks.

Although the HER-2 positive reports that I described here occurred in 2005, these types of misleading media reports are still happening today. Compounding this problem is access to the Internet, which most survivors have. There are many websites that contain erroneous and sometimes alarming information. Even legitimate websites that have the most scientifically vetted content may have chat rooms or other components where myths and other misinformation are presented as fact. Remember that the best medical advice that you will ever get about your specific diagnosis and treatment will come from your doctors and other members of your healthcare team.

When I counsel my patients, I warn them about what I call "emotional ambushes." These happen to everyone, but cancer survivors are particularly susceptible. What happens is pretty simple—you are in your usual state of mind, and you see or hear something that is not about you and doesn't affect your prognosis, but nevertheless your mood plummets and you being to worry about your own health. It may be a news report or something you read on the Internet or a well-meaning friend telling you a story about someone else who has cancer. The first step in dealing with an emotional ambush is to recognize it when it happens. You may certainly have empathy for other people when you hear a troubling story, but it's important to immediately recognize that this isn't about you and your health status hasn't changed. Recognizing an emotional ambush when it happens will help you to push away the worry and focus your attention on something more constructive.

Sometimes the setbacks really do affect you but aren't necessarily about your health or medical treatment. They may be just a matter of life getting in the way of healing. A rather dramatic and extremely upsetting setback of this kind happened to me the day after my first chemotherapy treatment. As I was getting used to the idea of feeling very sick physically, the phone rang. On the other end was my daughter's preschool teacher. I don't remember her exact words, but she said something like this: "I'm sorry to tell you this, but we let your daughter stir a cake mixture that has egg in it and she is having an allergic reaction." My youngest daughter has a life-threatening, anaphylactic type of allergy to egg, and I knew right away that this was going to be serious. I instructed the teacher to give her medication immediately, and I spent the rest of the day trying to control this allergic reaction. I rushed to her school, and by the time I got my daughter to the pediatrician, her face was so swollen it was almost unrecognizable. Trying to deal with my own illness on top of this crisis was overwhelming. But I had no choice.

Knowing that setbacks, both physical and emotional, are a normal and inevitable part of the recovery process can be reassuring. If you talk to long-term cancer survivors who are now thriving, it is unlikely that they will tell you, "During my treatment, everything went perfectly. There were no setbacks and I recovered easily, quickly, and completely." A tranquil and unblemished recovery is obviously what doctors work toward for their patients, but the reality is that few recoveries, whether from a life-threatening illness or from a minor injury, proceed in this manner. Instead, it is common to encounter obstacles that hinder and delay healing. However discouraging setbacks may be when you are in the midst of them, keep in mind that often setbacks, including cancer recurrence (in some instances), have little or nothing to do with your ultimate prognosis and life span. You can potentially experience many setbacks and still someday be one of those long-term cancer survivors who thrive.

Plateaus

Healing plateaus are also common during the recovery process. There are times when you haven't experienced a setback but neither do you seem to be making much progress. Patience and perspective are needed virtues for those of us who have been diagnosed with cancer. But it can be difficult to maintain these qualities during treatment and recovery. About one year after my last chemotherapy treatment, I had recovered a lot of my former strength, but I was still struggling with afternoon fatigue. Around 2:00 p.m. every day, I could count on feeling completely exhausted. This pattern went on for many months, and I knew I had hit a plateau in my recovery. Each morning I would awaken energized and looking forward to the day, and then I would become so exhausted that all I wanted to do was nap. I was sleeping well, eating a balanced and healthy diet, and generally feeling optimistic. I asked my doctor to run some tests to be sure that my thyroid gland was working properly and I wasn't anemic. Everything came back normal. So what was wrong? I had read quite a bit about cancer-related fatigue, and I knew that it could last well over one year. I often thought of Shakespeare's famous words, "How poor are they who have not patience. What wound did ever heal but by degrees?" Nevertheless, I was impatient. It had been long enough, and I was ready to feel good again—really good.

Around this time I began to push myself harder when I worked out. I increased the duration and intensity of my cardiovascular exercise program and added more weight and exercises to my strength-training routine. Whether it was these changes or just a matter of time (I think probably both played a role), over the next few months the afternoon exhaustion abated. It wasn't a sudden change, but one day I thought to myself, "I don't feel tired anymore in the afternoon."

I recognized my healing plateau, and I did what I routinely recommend to my patients—to check in with your doctor, describe your symptoms, follow through with any recommended tests, and continue to do the things that will ultimately facilitate healing.

Striving for Progress

Whenever you are not making progress in your recovery, whether it is physical or emotional or some of each, it is imperative that you talk to your doctor about your symptoms. Even if you are exceptionally well read or have a medical background, it is impossible for you to be objective. Moreover, as was the case with Dr. Cohn, there are likely gaps in your knowledge that only a physician who specializes in the kind of cancer that you have can fill.

Once active treatment ends, there may be long stretches between appointments with your oncologist. Furthermore, because the focus of your care for some weeks or months has been on the cancer, you may not have an appointment in the near future with your primary care physician. This posttreatment recovery period can feel a bit like a free fall, with no one guiding you.

If you are worried about any symptoms you are experiencing or you don't think you are making enough progress in healing, schedule an appointment to see both your primary care physician and your oncologist. Even if you aren't sure what to say or what is wrong, go and talk to them. It is likely that they have seen hundreds or thousands of patients in similar situations, and they will almost certainly be able to offer you practical advice geared for your particular circumstances.

In Table 14.1, I suggest some topics you might want to cover with your doctor and some wording to use. The reason I offer such specific suggestions is that some patients struggle to define what is really happening to them. They are in tune with their bodies, but trying to describe what is going on is not always easy. Dr. Cohn, who certainly had the medical vocabulary, explains what happened to him:

> The burden of having to deal with the problems of chemotherapy almost all the time depressed my emotional threshold. Frustrations stemming from situations beyond my control triggered outbursts of rage. Annoyances related to therapy included waiting for the results of blood tests in order to receive chemotherapy and the disappointment of not being able to convey to experts in oncology the expertise which I had acquired from being a chronic patient. Whether the failure of communication covered side-effects which had not been mentioned previously or the intensity of side-effects about which I had been told already, frustration still resulted. These feelings relate not only to medicine, however, but to the communication of any new experience.

Dr. Cohn is right. The language to describe any new experience doesn't exist for you until you have been through the experience and developed a description of it. Therefore, if you are not sure what to say or how to describe your physical or emotional state, you are like the rest of us. Just by showing up in your doctor's office, you communicate that something is troubling you enough to make the trip. Patients often go to their doctor without a clear explanation of why they are there. Most

Table 14.1. Things to Discuss with Your Doctor

I have been hearing things on the news about a new treatment for my type of cancer. Am I a candidate for this treatment? Are there any other treatments I should be considering?

I know that cancer prehabilitation and rehabilitation can help survivors to prepare for upcoming treatments and heal optimally. Do you think this will help me? May I have a referral to rehabilitation professionals that specialize in cancer?

I am experiencing pain on a daily basis that seems to be worse in the evening when I'm tired. The pain I am having is a general aching in my joints and low back. Is this normal? Should I have any tests done? What should I be doing to help alleviate this pain?

I awaken feeling refreshed, but my energy lags after lunch. I generally sleep well, but sometimes have difficulty falling asleep because I feel anxious about my future. Is this normal? Should I have any tests done? What can I be doing to feel more energetic?

Am I ready to exercise? Are there any precautions I should take? How much can I push myself?

I'd like to improve my diet. Can you recommend a dietician who is knowledgeable about my condition?

I have been feeling anxious, and I think that this is impacting my quality of life. I don't enjoy doing things that used to give me pleasure. I'd like some help with this. What do you suggest?

I have a tight feeling and some swelling over my surgical site. Is this normal?

What kind of testing do you think I should have in the future to monitor for a possible recurrence or progression of my cancer?

doctors are well schooled in asking questions that will get to the bottom of what is going on. What I am suggesting here is that if you have concerns, whether you can articulate them perfectly or not, make an appointment to see your doctor. Let her or him help you sort through what is happening to you. Use the suggestions in Table 14.1 to help guide you.

Keep in mind that it is normal and perfectly appropriate to want to be reassured by your doctor. If seeing your doctor provides a measure of reassurance and reduces some of the anxious feelings that you may be experiencing, going for an office visit is a perfectly healthy thing to do. Besides, your doctor may offer you important advice during this visit that you would not otherwise have obtained. Of course it doesn't make sense to go in every week for reassurance (if you find that you need this much help to alleviate anxious feelings, then you should see a mental health professional), but, for example, it is reasonable to schedule a follow-up appointment at the three-month mark instead of the six-month mark that your doctor suggested at your last visit. When physicians suggest follow-up appointment times to patients, they are usually giving them a general guideline about when would be a good time to come back. There are few hard and fast rules about follow-up appointments during the posttreatment phase, so if you have concerns, schedule a follow-up appointment sooner rather than later to address them.

REVISIT YOUR GOALS

Remember the ancient Chinese proverb, "A journey of a thousand miles begins with a single step"? By the time you read this book, you have come a long way on your journey. Not every step may have been sure footed, and at times you may have felt as if you weren't moving or were actually traveling backward, but almost certainly you have made tremendous progress. Pause now and reflect on how much you have accomplished in treating this illness and improving your physical health.

It is also helpful to periodically measure your progress by looking back at your goals. What were they? If you didn't accomplish every goal, consider what gains you have made. Depending on when you set your goals, it might be time to set some new ones or to modify your original objectives. If you didn't set any specific goals, perhaps now is the time to do it. Measuring your progress is a great way to maintain your perspective, even if there are bumps in the road.

REFERENCES

C. Kaelin, *Living through Breast Cancer* (New York: McGraw-Hill, 2005), p. 3.
K. Cohn, "Chemotherapy from an Insider's Perspective," *Lancet* 1 (1982): 1006–9.
J. Raymond and G. Cowley, "Targeting Tumors (Herceptin Cancer Treatment)," *Newsweek*, May 9, 2005, p. 13.

CHAPTER 15

LOOK WHAT'S ON
THE HORIZON

I always struggle with writing about future medical therapies, because although there is no doubt that further incredible advances in the treatment of cancer will occur, we cannot predict exactly what they will be. Since I first published this book, there have been numerous new advances to prevent oncological diseases from occurring in individuals at risk. For example, there is now a vaccine to prevent human papilloma virus (HPV) infection, which is responsible for some gynecological (cervical) cancers and head and neck cancers (through oral sex). Today, for most types of cancer it is still hard to predict who will develop which cancer and when. In the future, it is likely that doctors will be able predict what type of disease someone will contract and that they will be able to intervene *before* it develops. When prevention isn't possible, there will likely be cures that work in the same way that penicillin cures strep throat—easily, quickly, and with practically no toxicity to the patient (barring an allergic reaction to the drug, of course). And we can expect that researchers will develop a variety of measures that will work for different types of cancer.

The search for a cure for cancer, whether a vaccine or some other method, has been ongoing for many, many years. Cancer has been around for thousands of years. Before sophisticated imaging studies were done, however, it was not easily diagnosed, with the exception of some tumors that could be seen or felt such as those in the breast, until after the person died and an autopsy was done. For most of the time that cancer has existed, the treatments rendered have been completely ineffective. In the past, with the exception of the occasional surgical cure, cancer was essentially unstoppable.

The first real progress in the treatment of cancer, other than surgical advances, was the discovery of radiation and chemotherapy. Marie Curie is credited with discovering radiation, for which she received the Nobel Prize in physics in 1903, along with her husband. Scientists began to notice that radium crystals would damage skin cells and cause tumors to shrink. Although it would take years before doctors would understand exactly what was happening, during the first half of the twentieth century there was now a treatment, other than surgery, that could be tried on tumors. Ultimately scientists learned that radium is unstable at the atomic level and emits rays (called alpha, beta, and gamma) that, when focused on cells, cause the cells to change (become ionized) and disrupt their ability to divide (a process called *mitosis*). Since malignant cells are aberrant in that they divide more than normal cells (mitosis is not a controlled process in cancer cells; hence, the cells grow and spread, causing disease and ultimately death if not halted), they are particularly vulnerable to radiation, which affects this process. The right dose is essential, however. Too much radiation and all of the cells, normal and malignant, are killed. In a sad twist of fate, Marie Curie died in 1934 from radiation-induced leukemia because of overexposure to these potentially deadly rays. Too little radiation and the cancer cells aren't affected or are injured but are able to recover.

As I mentioned in the beginning of this book, chemotherapy can be traced to the discovery of nitrogen mustard as an effective treatment for cancer. In the 1940s a couple of scientists, Louis Goodman and Alfred Gilman, were recruited by the U.S. Department of Defense to examine the therapeutic value of a series of toxins that had been developed for use in chemical warfare. They knew from autopsies of soldiers unlucky enough to be exposed during World War I that mustard gas suppresses the lymphatic system. So they hypothesized that it might be a substance useful in treating lymphoma. Goodman and Gilman, who were both pharmacologists, convinced a thoracic surgeon colleague, Gustav Lindskog, to treat a patient who had non-Hodgkin's lymphoma with nitrogen mustard. As predicted, the tumors shrank, though unfortunately it was only a temporary regression. The principle of using chemotherapeutic drugs by injecting them into the body had been established, however. This bit of progress led to tremendous advances in treatment and cure rates for various cancers, including Hodgkin's lymphoma, which now is associated with extremely high cure rates when it is treated with a combination of chemotherapy and radiation.

By the mid-1970s many of the chemotherapeutic agents we use today had been synthesized. Significant advances have been made since then, though, in determining which medications should be used together, what doses are most effective, and what can be done to minimize side effects.

On the basis of these and other important scientific discoveries, people began to think that a cure for cancer was just around the corner. In his book on the history of breast cancer, James Olson writes:

> In the wake of World War II, and the success of the Manhattan Project in developing an atomic bomb, faith in science and technology spiked in American culture, and hope for a cure for cancer waxed just as strong. In what twenty-twenty hindsight sees as egregious hyperbole, news magazines and even some oncologists spoke of America's cancer-free future. According to a 1950 issue of *U.S. News and World Report*, "Millions of dollars, hundreds of scientists, and careful planning are being used in what authorities regard as medicine's counterpart of the wartime atom bomb project." In 1958, John Heller, head of the National Cancer Institute, remarked, "I've spent many years in cancer research. Now I believe that I will see the end of it." Such confidence, if unwarranted, was nevertheless rooted in real science and technology.

These overzealous predictions might seem foolish now, but keep in mind that this optimism about a cure for cancer came during the same time frame when antibiotics were becoming widely available, the polio vaccine was discovered, organ transplantation was found to be successful, and cardiac surgery became a viable option for people who would otherwise have had no hope of survival. Why shouldn't a cure for cancer be a realistic goal as well?

These cancer-cure predictions weren't as outrageous or wrong as they might appear at first glance, either. The official history of the American Cancer Society contains a fascinating chapter titled "Halfway to Victory." Here is an excerpt:

> In 1913 when the American Cancer Society was founded (as the American Society of the Control of Cancer), most physicians and nearly all patients believed that cancer was an incurable disease. Only a handful of doctors, mostly surgeons, rejected this nihilism, based on their experience, but there was no definition of cure for the disease, and no cure rate for any tumor. (The generally accepted definition of cancer cure today is no evidence of disease in a patient five years after the start of treatment, and a life expectancy equal to that of someone the same age who has never had cancer.)
>
> At the present time, for all serious tumors—excluding the nearly 100 percent curable skin cancers and *in situ* cancer of the uterine cervix—the relative survival rate of U.S. cancer patients for five years after diagnosis is 49 percent. . . . In other words, American biomedical science and medicine are about halfway to the goal of controlling cancer in human beings.

This book was published many years ago (in 1987), and the statistics are becoming more impressive every year. For some types of cancer, incredible progress has been made. Not long ago, I went to a cancer center that had a room in the back with two walls filled with pictures of children who had been treated there. I could tell from the clothing styles and the quality of the photos that one wall had been started many years ago while the other wall had photos of children who had been treated for cancer more recently. The nurse who was giving me a tour pointed to the older wall and said, "Most of these children are no longer with us." Then, she turned to the newer wall and said, "Due to advances in cancer treatment, we've been able to save the lives of the majority of these children." I looked at the two walls and thought about the huge advances that have been made in childhood cancers. Acute lymphoblastic leukemia used to be a uniformly fatal disease. When I first wrote this book, the cure rates were approaching 80 percent. Today, the cure rate is nearly 90 percent.

There has been tremendous progress with adult cancers, too. For example, during the 1970s, the five-year survival rate for breast cancer was approximately 75 percent and by the time you read this book it will be more than 90 percent. In women with early-stage breast cancer that has not spread to local tissues or distant organs, the survival rate is 99 percent. The past few years have demonstrated significant progress for women diagnosed with advanced breast cancer as well. The treatments are getting better and better and survival rates are increasing—regardless of the stage. This success in breast cancer has been due to many factors, including better treatments such as chemotherapy, hormone therapy, and targeted drugs.

Although advanced cancer is still the most challenging diagnosis for patients and doctors, progress is being made to treat, and sometimes cure, disease that has spread. In adults, testicular cancer, which can be cured even if it spreads, or metastasizes, to other organs, has an extremely high cure rate and is an amazing oncology success story. (Lance Armstrong recovered despite the fact that his testicular cancer spread to his lungs and his brain.) The same is true for Hodgkin's lymphoma. The ability to cure these advanced cancers, characterized by distant metastasis—a once (and often still) dreaded consequence of cancer because of its associated poor prognosis—is a forerunner of our future ability to cure all types of cancer, regardless of the stage.

Effective treatment for advanced cancer is one goal, but there are others as well. For example, biologic therapy and immunotherapy represent a more recent trend in cancer research (although the idea for this approach dates back at least several hundred years). Today immunotherapy is a highly promising area of cancer research. Vaccine research, which is included in this field, focuses on both the prevention and the treatment of cancer. Cancer is inextricably linked to the immune system, and we know that some viruses that people contract can lead to malignancy. For example, the hepatitis B virus is associated with liver cancer, the Epstein-Barr virus may be a factor in developing lymphoma, HPV (as I mentioned earlier) has a strong association with cervical as well as head and neck cancer, and the human immunodeficiency virus (HIV) is linked to Kaposi's sarcoma. Thus, it makes sense that developing vaccines would decrease the incidence of these types of cancer.

There is also a great deal of recent interest in therapies that can "target" specific components of malignant cells. The goal is to kill only the cancer cells and leave the normal cells intact. These are drugs or other substances that target specific molecules involved in malignant cell growth and survival. Some of the ways they may do this is by interfering with the tumor blood vessel development, by delivering toxic substances to the cells themselves, or by stimulating a person's own immune system to fight off the cancer cells. The concept of targeted therapy is so appealing because in the past the only option for chemotherapy was to kill all of the cells—normal and malignant. Increasingly, treatment regimens are becoming more individualized and taking into account specific markers that targeted drugs may be able to attack. We are already creating individualized treatments, often called *precision medicine,* and this approach will grow exponentially over the next few years as more and better targeted therapies become available.

Progress will also be made in diagnostic imaging studies, and other high-tech equipment will be improved, so that it will be possible to detect malignant cells much earlier than they can now be found. Early detection is crucial, and this will continue to be a prime focus of the fight against cancer. As will the focus on stopping cancer from developing in the first place. This is called *primary prevention* and involves recognizing the triggers that cause normal cells to become aberrant. For example, we know that exposure to the sun, nicotine use, and alcohol consumption may all make it more likely that a person will develop certain types of cancer. And, for those of us who have already had cancer, there is an emerging field that explores preventing cancer recurrence (often called *secondary prevention*). Throughout this book I have mentioned areas that look promising with respect to preventing cancer recurrence, such as diet and exercise (energetics).

Active research is going on in many other areas in the fight against cancer. The advances that have already been made in oncology and other subsets of medicine are tremendous and suggest that there is a legitimate reason to believe that cancer will someday become obsolete. Just as syphilologists (doctors who treat syphilis) have disappeared from the medical community, so will oncologists. Thus, while it is impossible to predict exactly what will happen with regard to eradicating this scourge, when people ask me if there will be a cure for cancer, I tell them the question is not if, but when.

It is possible that, for your type of cancer, there will be a break-through that may seem sudden but in reality is the fruit of many years of scientific exploration. In the meantime, you must focus on what you can control. Taking measures to improve your health in all the areas discussed in this book will help you to fight cancer or whatever other ill-nesses you are challenged with both now and in the future. What Helen Keller suggested so long ago is still true: "the world is full of suffering, but it is also full of the overcoming of it."

REFERENCES

J. S. Olson, *Bathsheba's Breast: Women, Cancer, and History* (Baltimore: Johns Hopkins University Press, 2002), p. 86.

W. S. Ross, Crusade: *The Official History of the American Cancer Society* (New York: Arbor House, 1987), p. 3.

American Cancer Society, *Cancer Treatment & Survivorship Facts & Figures 2014–2015*, p. 6. www.cancer.org/research/cancerfactsstatistics/survivor-facts-figures.

AFTERWORD

As I mentioned in the first chapter, the idea for this book came to me at an event to honor exceptional women. Seated beside me at the table was a woman who had been through cancer three times. The first time was in 1969 when she was 10 years old and diagnosed with Hodgkin's lymphoma. More than three decades later, she could still recall the pain in her chest where the doctors had operated to remove a tumor near her heart. The second cancer came when she was 30. She had flu-like symptoms, and a physician at Stanford Medical School told her that the lump in her neck, caused by thyroid cancer, was probably caused by the intensive radiation that she had undergone as a child. In 1998, cancer called a third time. This time it was in her breast. As I exchanged stories with this woman and other cancer survivors, I realized that there were things most of them could have done to achieve a quicker and easier recovery.

When I began to write this book, I knew that there were no scientific road maps that outlined a healing plan. Research studies are usually designed to answer a specific question, to test a particular hypothesis. They don't generate a plan that involves many components. So it is up to doctors, particularly those in primary care, oncology, and physical medicine and rehabilitation, to help patients understand what they need to do to physically and emotionally prepare for upcoming cancer treatments and to heal as well as possible once they have started.

I have created that road map specifically for cancer survivors, relying on the best scientific data as well as my many years of experience in helping people to heal from serious injuries and illnesses. I want you to have a true healing guide. The book does not take the place of your doctor's advice, of course, but rather is meant to give you additional information about important issues that may impact your recovery from cancer and its treatment. I encourage you to ask your doctor about cancer prehabilitation and rehabilitation. The professional help from experts in healing can be invaluable and should not be underestimated.

However, there are steps that you can take on your own at home as well. I suggest that you focus on three things initially: eating a healthy diet, exercising regularly, and resting well. There has never been a study investigating whether these core concepts are the most important in healing (though we have plenty of evidence looking at them individually to suggest that they are extremely important). Can you imagine a study in which one group of patients eats well, exercises regularly, and gets proper sleep, while another group eats junk food, doesn't exercise, and lacks sleep? The conclusion that the first group would thrive and heal much better is so obvious that no study will ever be done to prove this point.

Although the conclusion to such a fictitious study may be foregone, it is not always glaringly obvious exactly how you should improve in these areas to facilitate healing. It requires some thoughtful consideration, as I have suggested in the chapters that deal with these topics. And although diet, exercise, and rest are the main healing components, there are other important factors to consider during recovery: managing pain, recovering your emotional baseline, including spirituality in your healing plan if you are open to that concept, reaching out to your loved ones, and recognizing that setbacks are a part of the healing process.

By now you know that I have written from both my personal and professional experiences with cancer. Once when I went to an oncology follow-up appointment, the woman who checked me in told me that she had had stage 2 ovarian cancer seven years before. "It was the best thing that ever happened to me," she said. She went on to explain that previously she had been estranged from her adult daughter for many years, but, when she was diagnosed with cancer, they reconciled and have been close ever since.

Everyone is different, and we all integrate experiences in our own unique ways. The imprints that life's events leave on us are not all the same, even if the experience is similar. I never identified any favorable life-altering events associated with my cancer. What I saw when I was diagnosed with cancer and went through treatment was how it hurt me, my children, my husband, my mother and my siblings, my friends, and my patients. For me, physically healing was important not only to regain my strength but to put cancer in its place. To say that healing physically eliminated the emotional toll that cancer took would not be accurate. But the more I healed physically, the better I felt in body and spirit. The same is true for many cancer survivors.

When I began my recovery, I made lists of my goals, and I made lists of what I needed to do to accomplish my goals. I am admittedly fond of lists, because they help to give me the perspective I need to do what I want to do. Before long, I abandoned my lists; I didn't need them anymore. The lifestyle changes that I have written about in this book became so much a part of my life that I no longer needed to write them down. Still, I do like lists. I often think of this when I hear the country singer, Toby Keith, sing this lyric: "Start livin'—that's the next thing on my list."

WHERE TO FIND HELP

GENERAL RESOURCES

ABCD: After Breast Cancer Diagnosis
5775 N. Glen Park Road, Suite 201
Glendale, WI 53209
800-977-4121
(Breast Cancer Helpline—Immediate Support from a Survivor & Mentor Match, 414-977-1780)
www.afterbreastcancerdiagnosis.com

American Cancer Society
1599 Clifton NE
Atlanta, GA 30329
800-ACS-2345 (800-227-2345)
www.cancer.org
  The ACS is a nationwide community-based volunteer health organization. The goal of the organization is to eliminate cancer as a major health problem by preventing the disease, saving lives, and diminishing suffering through research, education, advocacy, and service. The ACS offers many programs. The website has sections for patients, families and friends, survivors, donors and volunteers, and professionals.

Breastcancer.org
111 Forrest Avenue
Narbeth, PA 19072
610-664-1990
www.breastcancer.org
  Breastcancer.org is a nonprofit organization that provides information about breast cancer. In order to facilitate the decision-making process,

breastcancer.org helps women and their families make sense of complex medical and personal information about breast cancer. In addition to information about prevention, symptoms and diagnosis, treatment, recovery, and support, the website offers monthly online conferences with breast cancer experts and monthly reports on breakthroughs in breast cancer research.

CancerNet
www.cancernet.gov

CancerNet is a comprehensive website that contains information on diagnosis, treatment, support, resources, literature, clinical trials, prevention and risk factors, and testing. Publications can be ordered online (publications.nci.nih.gov). Some publications are available in Spanish.

Cancer Support Community
1050 17th Street NW, Suite 500
Washington, DC 20036
202-659-9709
888-793-9355
www.cancersupportcommunity.org

The Cancer Support Community is dedicated to providing support, education and hope to people affected by cancer. In 2009, the Wellness Community and Gilda's Club Worldwide joined forces to become the Cancer Support Community. By helping to complete the cancer care plan, this organization optimizes patient care by providing essential but often overlooked services, including support groups, counseling, education and healthy lifestyle programs. Today, the Cancer Support Community provides the high quality emotional and social support through a large network.

CancerTrials
http://www.cancer.gov/clinicaltrials

This site offers information about ongoing cancer clinical trials and an explanation of what a trial is.

Leukemia and Lymphoma Society
1311 Mamaroneck Avenue
White Plains, NY 10605
800-955-4572
914-949-5213
www.leukemia-lymphoma.org

The LLS, formerly the Leukemia Society of America, is a national health agency that seeks cures for leukemia, lymphoma, Hodgkin's disease, and myeloma. The local chapters of the LLS also help patients and their families improve their quality of life by offering programs and resources that include financial assistance, support groups, patient education and information, and referrals to local resources.

Livestrong Foundation
2201 E. Sixth Street
Austin, TX 78702
855-220-7777
www.livestrong.org
   Livestrong provides practical information for cancer survivors.

Look Good . . . Feel Better
800-395-LOOK (800-395-5665)
www.lookgoodfeelbetter.org
   Look Good . . . Feel Better is a free public-service program that teaches patients with cancer techniques to enhance their appearance and self-image during chemotherapy and radiation.

National Cancer Institute
800-4-CANCER (800-422-6237)
www.cancer.gov
   This government agency provides information on cancer research, diagnosis, and treatment. People with cancer, caregivers, and health care professionals can call the toll-free number for cancer-related information, including information about complementary and alternative medicine and nutrition in cancer care. Spanish-speaking staff and Spanish materials are available.

National Coalition for Cancer Survivorship
1010 Wayne Avenue, Suite 315
Silver Spring, MD 20910
877-NCCS-YES (877-622-7937)
www.canceradvocacy.org
   The NCCS is a survivor-led advocacy organization for cancer survivorship and support. The NCCS focuses on educating people affected by cancer and speaking about issues related to cancer care. The website has links to online cancer resources, support groups, and survivorship programs; a newsletter; and a self-help audio program that coaches people with cancer on meeting the challenges of their illness.

National Comprehensive Cancer Network

275 Commerce Drive, Suite 300

Fort Washington, PA 19034

215-690-0300

www.nccn.org

The NCCN is a nonprofit, membership organization that is an alliance of cancer centers. The American Cancer Society and the NCCN have translated the NCCN Clinical Practice Guidelines into a patient-friendly resource. The guidelines offer easy-to-understand information for patients and family members about treatment options for each stage of cancer. The patient-friendly guidelines are available for breast, prostate, lung, colon, and rectal cancer and for nausea and vomiting, fever and neutropenia, cancer-related fatigue, and cancer pain. Additional guidelines are in development.

National Library of Medicine

8600 Rockville Pike

Bethesda, MD 20894

888-FIND-NLM (888-346-3656)

www.nlm.nih.gov

The NLM collects, organizes, and makes available health information. Both health professionals and the public use its electronic databases extensively throughout the world. Materials are available in multiple languages.

SHARE (Self-Help for Women with Breast or Ovarian Cancer)

1501 Broadway, Suite 704A

New York, NY 10036

866-891-2392 (breast cancer toll-free)

212-382-2111 (breast cancer hotline)

212-719-1204 (ovarian cancer hotline)

212-719-4454 (Spanish hotline)

www.sharecancersupport.org

SHARE is a self-help organization for women and men who have been affected by breast or ovarian cancer. Volunteers who have survived breast or ovarian cancer staff the various hotlines. The volunteers and the website offer information about cancer, printed materials, and referrals to national organizations.

Survivorship A to Z

www.survivorshipatoz.org

Survivorship A to Z offers financial, legal, and practical information for cancer survivors. The organization provides tools to help make complicated decisions more simple for survivors. For example, they might assist in deciding how to choose among health insurance policies from the point of view of a person with a cancer diagnosis, or how to complete forms such as the Social Security Disability Insurance application.

Susan G. Komen
5005 LBJ Freeway, Suite 250
Dallas, TX 75244
877-GO-KOMEN (877-465-6636)
www.komen.org
Susan G. Komen funds research grants and supports education, screening, and treatment projects in communities around the world. In addition to information about breast cancer, the website contains information about obtaining grants, making donations, participating in events, subscribing to free newsletters, and purchasing gifts and educational materials from the Foundation.

Young Survival Coalition
80 Broad Street, Suite 1700
New York, NY 10004
877-972-1011
www.youngsurvival.org
Women under the age of 40 who were breast cancer survivors founded Young Survival Coalition. The main goal of the coalition is to educate health care providers and the public about how breast cancer impacts younger women. The website offers information about breast cancer, as well as links to relevant resources.

Resources for Cancer Rehabilitation
American Academy of Physical Medicine and Rehabilitation (for locating physiatrists)
9700 W. Bryn Mawr Avenue, Suite 200
Rosemont, IL 60018-5701
847-737-6000
847-737-6001 (fax)
info@aapmr.org
www.aapmr.org
The American Academy of Physical Medicine and Rehabilitation is the national medical society representing more than 7,500 physicians (physiatrists) who are specialists in the field of physical medicine and rehabilitation.

American Congress of Rehabilitation Medicine (ACRM)

11654 Plaza America Drive, Suite 535

Reston, VA 20190

703-435-5335

866-692-1619 (fax)

info@ACRM.org

www.acrm.org

The American Congress of Rehabilitation Medicine (ACRM) is a professional association representing all members of the interdisciplinary rehabilitation team, including physicians, psychologists, rehabilitation nurses, occupational therapists, physical therapists, speech therapists, recreation specialists, case managers, rehabilitation counselors, vocational counselors, and disability management specialists.

American Occupational Therapy Association, Inc.

4720 Montgomery Lane, Suite 200

Bethesda, MD 20814-3449

800-377-8555

301-652-6611

301-652-7711 (fax)

www.aota.org

The American Occupational Therapy Association (AOTA) is a national professional association that represents the interests and concerns of occupational therapy practitioners and students of occupational therapy and strives to improve the quality of occupational therapy services.

American Physical Therapy Association

1111 N. Fairfax Street

Alexandria, VA 22314-1488

800-999-APTA (800-999-2782)

703-684-7343 (fax)

memberservices@apta.org

www.apta.org

The American Physical Therapy Association (APTA) is a national professional organization including more than 72,000 members. The organization represents and promotes the profession of physical therapy and strives to further the profession's role in the prevention, diagnosis, and treatment of movement dysfunctions and the enhancement of the physical health and functional abilities of members of the public. Its goal is to foster advancements in physical therapy through practice, research, and education.

American Speech-Language-Hearing Association

2200 Research Boulevard

Rockville, MD 20850-3289

301-296-5700

301-296-8580 (fax)

actioncenter@asha.org

www.asha.org

The American Speech-Language-Hearing Association (ASHA) is the professional, scientific, and credentialing association of more than 130,000 members and affiliates who are audiologists; speech-language pathologists; and speech, language, and hearing scientists.

Council of State Administrators of Vocational Rehabilitation

1 Research Court, Suite 450

Rockville, MD 20850

301-519-8023

301-654-8414

www.rehabnetwork.org

The mission of the Council is to maintain and enhance a national program of public vocational rehabilitation services so that individuals with disabilities can achieve employment, economic self-sufficiency, independence, and inclusion and integration into the community. They provide counseling and other support services to help people find jobs.

National Lymphedema Network

225 Bush Street, Suite 357

San Francisco, CA 94104

800-541-3259 (hotline)

415-908 -3681

www.lymphnet.org

The NLN is an internationally recognized nonprofit organization that provides education and guidance to lymphedema patients, health care professionals, and the general public. The NLN supports research into the causes and possible alternative treatments for this condition. The website offers information about lymphedema treatment centers, health care professionals, training programs, and support groups.

STAR Program

www.oncologyrehabpartners.com

STAR Program certification (Survivorship Training and Rehabilitation) provides hospitals, cancer centers and group practices with the tools they need to deliver high-quality cancer rehabilitation care. STAR Programs consist of multidisciplinary rehabilitation service lines that improve patient care and outcomes. To find a STAR Program near you, visit the Oncology Rehab Partners' website.

RESOURCES FOR FAMILIES, CHILDREN, AND PARTNERS

American Association for Marriage and Family Therapy (AAMFT)

112 S. Alfred Street

Alexandria, VA 22314-3061

703-838-9808

703-838-9805 (fax)

www.aamft.org

The American Association for Marriage and Family Therapy (AAMFT) is a professional association for the field of marriage and family therapy. AAMFT provides referrals to local marriage and family therapists. They also provide educational materials to help couples live with illness and other issues related to families and health.

American Association of Pastoral Counselors

9504A Lee Highway

Fairfax, VA 22031-2302

703-385-6967

www.aapc.org

The American Association of Pastoral Counselors offers an online directory of Certified Pastoral Counselors across the country, as well as links to other relevant resources.

American Association of Sexuality Educators, Counselors, and Therapists

1444 I Street NW, Suite 700

Washington, DC 20005

202-449-1099

www.aasect.org

The AASECT is a nonprofit, interdisciplinary professional organization that promotes understanding of human sexuality and healthy sexual behavior. In addition to sex educators, sex counselors, and sex therapists, AASECT members include physicians, nurses, social workers, psychologists, allied health professionals, clergy members, lawyers, sociologists, marriage and family planning specialists, and researchers, as well as students in relevant professional disciplines. The website offers information for the public and professionals, with links to a variety of related organizations.

American Childhood Cancer Organization

10920 Connecticut Avenue, Suite A

Kensington, MD 20985

855-858-2226

301-962-3520

www.acco.org

Candlelighters is a nonprofit organization that educates, supports, serves, and advocates for families of children with cancer and survivors of childhood cancer, as well as the health care professionals who care for children with cancer. The ACCF website provides information on events, treatment, support, and advocacy. It also has a section specifically for children.

American Society for Reproductive Medicine

1209 Montgomery Highway

Birmingham, AL 35216-2809

205-978-5000

www.asrm.org

The ASMR is a multidisciplinary society for health care professionals who are interested in or practice reproductive medicine. In addition to offering professionals the latest updates in reproductive medicine, the website provides information on continuing medical education, links to other resources, and subscription information for the society's peer-reviewed journal. There is also a section for the public that includes information about fertility.

Cancer Care, Inc.

275 Seventh Avenue

New York, NY 10001

800-813-HOPE (800-813-4673)

212-712-8400

www.cancercare.org

www.cancercare.org/espanol (Spanish version)

Cancer Care, Inc., is a nonprofit social service agency that offers counseling and guidance to help patients and their families and friends cope with cancer. The website provides information on specific cancers and treatment, clinical trials, and links to other sites. The organization also supplies videos, support groups, workshops, seminars and clinics, a newsletter, and other publications. A Spanish-speaking staff is available.

Caregiver Action Network

2000 M Street NW, Suite 400

Washington, DC 20036

202-772-5050

www.caregiveraction.org

info@caregiveraction.org

The NFCA provides education, support, and advocacy for family caregivers. The website offers publications and other materials for purchase, as well as some free, downloadable information. There are also links to other websites that provide information about specific diseases and disabilities and other health care issues.

CDC Reproductive Health Information Source

Division of Reproductive Health

National Center for Chronic Disease Prevention and Health Promotion

Centers for Disease Control and Prevention

1600 Clifton Road

Atlanta, GA 30329-4027

770-488-5200

www.cdc.gov/reproductivehealth/

This division of the Centers for Disease Control and Prevention focuses on how to best keep women reproductively healthy, through both research and practical measures. The website offers information to professionals and the public about the latest trends and breakthroughs in reproductive medicine, with relevant links to both federal and nonfederal organizations.

Kids Konnected

26071 Merit Circle, Suite 103

Laguna Hills, CA 92653

800-899-2866

949-582-5443

www.kidskonnected.org

Kids Konnected, a national nonprofit organization, offers groups and programs for children who have a parent with cancer. In addition to answering questions and providing support to children, the organization offers an information packet of books and other information, referrals to local support groups, a quarterly newsletter for children, summer camps, socials, and grief workshops.

Livestrong Fertility

2201 E. Sixth Street

Austin, Texas 78702

888-994-HOPE (888-994-4673)

www.livestrong.org/we-can-help/fertility-services

The Well Spouse Association

63 W. Main Street, Suite H

Freehold, NJ 07728

800-838-0879

www.wellspouse.org

info@wellspouse.org

Well Spouse is a national not-for-profit membership organization that offers support to wives, husbands, and partners of the chronically ill or disabled. Well Spouse support groups meet monthly. The website provides information about how to become a member, meeting times and places, activities, conferences, printed material, and links to other relevant organizations.

RESOURCES TO FIND HEALTH CARE PROFESSIONALS

American Medical Association

AMA Plaza

330 N. Wabash Avenue, Suite 39300

Chicago, IL 60611-5885

800-621-8335

www.ama-assn.org

The AMA, the country's largest physicians' group, develops and promotes standards in medical practice, research, and education. The consumer health information section on the association's website has databases on physicians and hospitals that can be searched by medical specialty, as well as information on specific conditions.

American Society of Clinical Oncology

2318 Mill Road, Suite 800

Alexandria, VA 22314

888-651-3038

571-483-1780

www.asco.org

www.cancer.net (patient website)

The ASCO is an international professional organization representing more than 23,000 cancer specialists involved in clinical research, advocacy, and patient care. The ASCO Cancer.net website, with support from the Conquer Cancer Foundation, offers cancer patients, doctors, and researchers information on defining, understanding, and coping with cancer, as well as news and information about drug treatments, cancer legislation, and links to related sites.

RESOURCES FOR COMPLEMENTARY THERAPIES AND NUTRITION

Academy of Nutrition and Dietetics

120 S. Riverside Plaza, Suite 2000
Chicago, IL 60606-6995
800-877-1600
www.eatright.org

The ADA, the world's largest organization of food and nutrition professionals, promotes nutrition, health, and well-being. The website has information on diet and nutrition and publications, as well as a registered dietitian locator service, which includes dietitians who specialize in cancer nutrition.

Consortium of Academic Health Centers for Integrative Medicine

www.imconsortium.org

The Consortium of Academic Health Centers for Integrative Medicine includes twenty-seven academic medical centers. The consortium's mission is to transform medicine and health care through scientific studies, new models of clinical care, and educational programs that integrate biomedicine, the complexity of human beings, the intrinsic nature of healing, and diverse therapeutic systems. Its goal is to make a difference in people's health by advocating an integrative model of health care that incorporates mind, body, and spirit.

Harvard School of Public Health

Department of Nutrition
665 Huntington Avenue
Boston, MA 02115
617-432-1851
www.hsph.harvard.edu/nutritionsource/

The Nutrition Source is a website that is maintained by the Department of Nutrition at the Harvard School of Public Health. The website serves as a resource for the most up-to-date information on diet and nutrition and dispels rumors and fallacies about fad diets.

The Interactive Healthy Eating Index

http://www.cnpp.usda.gov/healthyeatingindex

The Interactive Healthy Eating Index is an online dietary assessment tool developed by the USDA's Center for Nutrition Policy and Promotion. The website has downloadable publications and data files.

Meals on Wheels Association of America

413 N. Lee Street

Alexandria, VA 22314

888-998-6325

www.mowaa.org

Meals on Wheels is a membership association that offers programs to provide home-delivered and group meals. The organization aims to improve the quality of life of those who need assistance. Some programs may provide other health and social services.

Memorial Sloan-Kettering Cancer Center

About Herbs

www.mskcc.org/mskcc/html/11570.cfm

The About Herbs website provides information for health care professionals and consumers about herbs, botanicals, and other supplements, as well as alternative or unproven cancer therapies, including details about adverse effects, interactions, and potential benefits or problems.

National Center for Complementary and Alternative Medicine

National Institutes of Health

9000 Rockville Pike

Bethesda, MD 20892

888-644-6226

866-464-3613 (TTY)

301-231-7537, ext. 5 (from outside the U.S.)

866-464-3616 (fax)

http://nccam.nih.gov

The NCCAM explores complementary and alternative healing practices through research, research training and education, outreach, and integration. The NCCAM website offers publications, information for researchers, frequently asked questions, and links to other complementary and alternative medicine–related resources. The NCCAM Clearinghouse is the public's source for scientifically based information on CAM and for information about NCCAM.

National Heart, Lung, and Blood Institute Health Information Center
P.O. Box 30105
Bethesda, MD 20824-0105
301-592-8573
www.nhlbi.nih.gov/health/educational/wecan/healthy-weight-basics/body-mass-index.htm (body mass index calculator)

This website provides information about the body mass index and what constitutes a healthy weight for both men and women. The website also provides links to information about controlling food and planning menus.

Quackwatch, Inc.
P.O. Box 1747
Allentown, PA 18105
610-437-1795
www.quackwatch.com

Quackwatch is a nonprofit corporation that exposes and combats health-related frauds, myths, fads, and fallacies. Its primary focus is on quackery-related information that is difficult or impossible to get elsewhere. The website contains links to information on publications for sale; general observations; questionable products, services, and theories; questionable advertisements; nonrecommended sources of health advice; consumer protection; consumer strategy (health promotion, tips for provider selection, and disease management); education for consumers and health professionals; research projects; legal and political activities; and other recommended links.

USDA Food and Nutrition Information Center
National Agricultural Library, Room 108
10301 Baltimore Avenue
Beltsville, MD 20705-2351
301-504-5719
301-504-5414 (for inquiries to dietitians and nutritionists)
http://fnic.nal.usda.gov/

The USDA's FNIC is an information center for the National Agricultural Library. FNIC materials and services include dietitians and nutritionists available to answer inquiries, publications on food and nutrition, and resource lists and bibliographies. The FNIC website includes information on dietary supplements, food safety, dietary guidelines, food composition facts (including fast food), a list of available publications, and information on popular topics.

U.S. Food and Drug Administration

10903 New Hampshire Avenue
Silver Spring, MD 20993
888-INFO-FDA (888-463-6332)
www.fda.gov

The FDA is a public health agency that enforces the Federal Food, Drug, and Cosmetic Act and other laws, promotes health by helping safe and effective products reach the market in a timely manner, and monitors products for continued safety once they are in use. The website has information on FDA-regulated products.

Resources for Pain Management

American Academy of Pain Medicine

8735 W. Higgins Road, Suite 300
Chicago, IL 60631-2738
847-375-4731
www.painmed.org

The American Academy of Pain Medicine is the medical specialty society for physicians practicing pain medicine. The academy is involved in education, training, advocacy, and research in pain medicine. The AAPM website has links to other sites related to pain and pain medicine and also features membership information and links to the academy's publications and products.

American Chronic Pain Association

P.O. Box 850
Rocklin, CA 95677
800-533-3231
www.theacpa.org
acpa@pacbell.net

The American Chronic Pain Association offers information and support for people with chronic pain and their families. The ACPA also strives to raise awareness among people in the medical profession, policymakers, and the general public about living with chronic pain. The website has some free downloadable information about managing pain, as well as an online store where videos, manuals, and other materials can be purchased.

American Pain Society

8735 W. Higgins Road, Suite 300
Chicago, IL 60631
847-375-4715
www.ampainsoc.org
info@ampainsoc.org

The American Pain Society, a nonprofit membership organization of scientists, clinicians, policy analysts, and others, seeks to advance pain-related research, education, treatment, and professional practice. The website provides some publications on pain, which can either be viewed online or ordered for a fee.

MENTAL HEALTH RESOURCES

American Association for Marriage and Family Therapy

112 S. Alfred Street
Alexandria, VA 22314-3061
703-838-9808
www.aamft.org

The AAMFT is the professional organization for marriage and family therapists. In addition to resources for professionals, the organization provides the public with referrals to marriage and family therapists. It also supplies educational materials on living with illness and other issues related to families and health.

American Counseling Association

5999 Stevenson Avenue
Alexandria, VA 22304-3300
800-347-6647
703-823-0252
www.counseling.org

The ACA is a nonprofit professional and educational organization that supports the counseling profession. The website has information for students, consumers, and counselors.

American Psychiatric Association

1000 Wilson Boulevard, Suite 1825
Arlington, VA 22209-3901
888-35-PSYCH (888-357-7924)
www.psych.org

The American Psychiatric Association is a medical specialty society. The more than 35,000 U.S. and international physicians belonging to the APA work together to provide humane care and effective treatment for anyone with mental disorders, including mental retardation and substance-related disorders. The website includes information about the APA and links to related organizations.

American Psychological Association

750 First Street NE
Washington, DC 20002-4242
800-374-2721
202-336-6123 (TDD/TTY)
www.apa.org

The American Psychological Association offers referrals to psychologists in local areas and provides information on family issues, parenting, and health. Its website has links to state psychological associations that may also provide local referrals.

American Psychosocial Oncology Society (APOS)

154 Hansen Road, Suite 201
Charlottesville, VA 22911
866-276-7443
434-293-5350
434-977-1856 (fax)
info@apos-society.org
http://www.apos-society.org

The American Psychosocial Oncology Society focuses on methods to enhance the recognition and treatment of psychological, social, behavioral, and spiritual aspects of cancer. They provide clinical information, education, and a hotline for counseling and support services in order to promote the well-being of patients with cancer and families at all stages of disease. They also focus on raising the level of awareness of health professionals and the public about psychological, social, behavioral, and spiritual domains of care for patients with cancer.

National Association of Social Workers

750 First Street NE, Suite 700
Washington, DC 20002-4241
202-408-8600
www.socialworkers.org

The National Association of Social Workers is the world's largest membership organization of professional social workers. The NASW enhances the professional growth and development of its members, creates and maintains professional standards, and advances sound social policies. The website has information and links for professionals and the general public. The NASW's publications can be ordered online for a fee.

AARP

601 E Street NW
Washington, DC 20049
888-OUR-AARP (888-687-2277)
www.aarp.org
www.aarphealthcare.com/health-discounts/prescription-discounts.html
(pharmacy service)

The AARP is a nonprofit membership organization open to anyone 50 years old or older. Its member services include information on managed and long-term care, Medicare, and Medicaid. The website has information on a pharmacy service that offers discounts on drugs used for cancer treatment and pain relief.

Americans with Disability Act (ADA)

800-514-0301
800-514-0383 (TTY)
www.ada.gov

This service employs specialists who can answer questions about the Americans with Disabilities Act (ADA) and provide information about the programs and services available through state and local governments. The website has a list of free booklets and publications you can order or read online. Many of these publications are available in languages other than English.

NeedyMeds

P.O. Box 219
Gloucester, MA 01931
800-503-6897
978-281-6666
206-260-8850
info@needymeds.org
www.needymeds.com

The mission of NeedyMeds is to be the best source of accurate, comprehensive, and up-to-date information on programs that assist people in paying for medications and health care, and in helping people apply to those programs. NeedyMeds also provides health education. NeedyMeds is not a patient assistance program, but rather a source of information on thou-

280   { APPENDIX }

sands of programs that may be able to offer assistance to people in need. NeedyMeds offers a free drug discount card that may help patients obtain a substantially lower price on their medications. This card can be used instead of insurance or by anyone without insurance.

Partnership for Prescription Assistance

888-4PPA-NOW (888-477-2669)

www.pparx.org

The Partnership for Prescription Assistance helps qualifying patients without prescription drug coverage get the medicines they need through the program that is right for them. The organization provides a directory of prescription drug patient assistance programs that contains information about how to make a request for assistance, what prescription medicines are covered, and basic eligibility criteria.

INDEX

AARP, 280
abandonment, 180, 202, 203, 217
ABCD: After Breast Cancer Diagnosis, 263
Academy of Nutrition and Dietetics, 274
acetaminophen, 164
acupuncture, 71–74, 78, 85, 87–89, 90, 172, 192
Adriamycin, 101
advocacy organizations, 263, 265, 271–74, 277. *See also* resources
aerobic (cardiovascular) exercise, 50, 99, 101, 106–8, 111, 113, 153, 167, 191, 248; target heart rate for, 104
After Breast Cancer (Schnipper), 227
alcohol, 2, 52, 128, 130, 134–36, 137, 153, 192, 222, 257; opioids and, 159; self-medicating with, 135–36, 187; sleep and, 144, 150
The Almost Effect, 189
alternative therapies. *See* complementary and alternative medicine
American Academy of Pain Medicine, 277
American Academy of Physical Medicine and Rehabilitation, 68, 267
American Association for Marriage and Family Therapy, 270, 278
American Association of Pastoral Counselors, 270
American Association of Sexuality

Educators, Counselors, and Therapists, 270
American Cancer Society (ACS), 2, 16–17, 90, 108, 131, 134, 238, 255, 263, 266
American Childhood Cancer Organization, 271
American Chronic Pain Association, 277
American College of Sports Medicine, 94, 100
American Congress of Rehabilitation Medicine, 268
American Counseling Association, 278
American Dietetic Association, 131
American Heart Association, 100
American Medical Association, 82, 86, 273
American Occupational Therapy Association, Inc., 268
American Pain Society, 278
American Physical Therapy Association, 100, 268
American Psychiatric Association, 278–79
American Psychological Association, 279
American Psychosocial Oncology Society, 279
American Psychosomatic Society, 214
American Society for Reproductive Medicine, 271

283

American Society of Clinical Oncology, 273–74
American Speech-Language-Hearing Association, 269
Americans with Disabilities Act (ADA), 280
amitriptyline (Elavil), 186
Anafranil (clomipramine), 186
The Anatomy of Hope (Groopman), 205
Ancoli-Israel, Sonia, 144
anemia, 101, 127, 137, 141, 142, 143, 149, 151, 152, 187, 220
anger, 83, 174, 179, 180, 189, 191, 225
anti-anxiety medications, 182, 185, 188, 190, 221
antidepressants, 185–87, 188, 190, 191, 194, 221; for pain, 160, 164, 165; side effects of, 186
anti-inflammatory medications, 158, 164, 165
antioxidants, 10, 25, 123–25, 145
antiseizure drugs, 158, 164
anxiety/worry, 17, 22, 65, 69, 174, 178, 181–82, 187–89, 194, 211; alcohol and, 187; CAM therapies for, 83, 85, 87, 167; about cancer recurrence, 184; about children, 227, 228, 229, 232, 234; about diet, 118, 121; due to emotional ambushes, 246; exercise for, 94, 97; about future, 6, 30–31, 179, 181; about infertility, 225; intimacy and, 219, 220, 221; journaling for, 194; medications for, 182, 185, 188, 190, 221; physical changes causing, 185, 188; psychological therapy for, 171, 182, 190; in PTSD, 191; recovery and, 27, 182–83; sleep and, 137, 139, 140, 141, 143, 144, 146, 148, 149, 154, 183; spirituality and, 196, 198, 199, 200, 208; support groups and, 237, 238; symptoms of, 182; talking to doctor about, 187, 189, 249, 250–51
appetite changes, 7, 120, 138, 160, 161, 180, 183, 188, 191; in children, 234
appreciation, 30, 203, 209, 218
Armstrong, Lance, 256
arthritis, 45, 73, 85, 87, 104, 113, 143, 163, 166, 169, 170

Audette, Joseph, 88
Ayurvedic medicine, 6, 76, 78–79

back pain, 45, 73, 90, 97, 110–11, 113, 161–62, 163, 165, 169
Baima, Jennifer, 98
Bald in the Land of Big Hair (Rodgers), 216
Ball, Thomas, 151–52
bathing/showering, 47–48, 56, 150
Bathsheba's Breast (Olson), 85
behavioral changes, 180; in children, 232–33
Bennett, Arnold, 39
Benson, Herbert, 211
biomarkers, 23
bisphosphonates, 160
bladder cancer, 123
blood cell counts, 102, 116, 151
blood pressure, 102, 156, 189; CAM therapies and, 81, 83, 207; drug-induced elevation of, 160, 164, 186; high, 113; medications for, 104, 221; stress and, 211
blood sugar: diet and, 125, 137, 154; exercise and, 96, 97, 113
blood tests, 152, 249
body image, 219
body mass index (BMI), 105
body mechanics, 53
bone cancer, 160–61
bone health, 127–28, 168; exercise for, 96, 97, 109, 113, 128; fractures, 14, 82, 127, 160; osteopenia/osteoporosis, 82, 83, 88, 113, 127–28
bone mineral density, 127
botanicals, 80–81
botulinum toxin injections, 165, 166
Bowling Alone (Putnam), 239
brachytherapy, 21
Bradshaw, Terry, 45
breast cancer, 9, 17, 22, 24, 49, 167, 259; alcohol and, 134, 135; CAM treatments for, 84, 85–86; choosing right treatment for, 66–67; crisis of diagnosis of, 31; diet and, 98, 123; emotional impact of, 184–85; exercise and, 61–62, 95–96, 112;

fatigue and, 139, 152; fertility and, 225; health food store recommendations and, 89–90; HER-2 positive, 245–46; history of, 85–86, 216, 252, 254; journaling and, 193; lumpectomy for, 184, 244; lymphedema after surgery for, 114, 171–72; mastectomy for, 7, 17, 89, 112, 165, 185, 215, 238, 244; pain management in, 167, 171; parenting and, 227; prognosis for, 9, 177, 180–81, 245–46; psychosocial support and outcome of, 214–15, 217; resources for, 263–64, 266, 267; setbacks in recovery from, 243–44; sexuality and, 219; spirituality/religion and, 196, 199, 203, 204; support groups for, 237, 238; survival rate for, 9, 255–56

Breast Cancer Awareness Month, 31

Breastcancer.org, 263–64

breath-focused meditation, 209

Brehony, Kathleen, 239

Brenner, Paul, 90

Brothers, Joyce, 178

Buddha in the Waiting Room (Brenner), 90

Buddhism, 83, 204, 206, 208, 209

bupropion (Wellbutrin), 186

bursitis injections, 165, 166

caffeine, 128, 150

calcium supplements, 127–28, 130

caloric intake, 119, 137, 234

Campbell, Joseph, 14

Cancer Care, Inc., 271

cancer cells, 1, 17–18; therapy targeting, 5, 19, 20, 21, 256–57; treatment effects on, 5, 19, 20, 253

Cancer in the Family, 228

CancerNet, 264

Cancer Schmancer (Drescher), 184

Cancer Support Community, 211, 264

CancerTrials, 264

cannabinoids, 161

carbohydrates, 119, 120, 125–26, 137

carcinogens in diet, 126

cardiac stress test, 101, 102

cardiovascular (aerobic) exercise, 50,

99, 101, 106–8, 111, 113, 153, 167, 191, 248; target heart rate for, 104

Caregiver Action Network, 272

Carli, Franco, 98–99

Carter, Jimmy, 217–18

Cassileth, Barrie, 70–71

Catholicism, 204, 206

Celexa (citalopram), 186

cell growth, 17–18

Centers for Disease Control and Prevention (CDC), 105

Centers for Disease Control and Prevention, Reproductive Health Information Source, 272

cervical cancer, 169, 225, 252, 256

chemo brain, 148–50

chemotherapy, 3, 19; dose-dense regimen of, 44; exercise and, 102; history of, 253–54; targeted drugs for, 5; toxicity of, 44

chi, 71–72, 78

children of cancer patient, 215, 226–35; adolescent child, 231–32; answering questions about death, 229; appetite changes in, 234; behavioral changes in, 233; caring for, 4–5, 42, 217, 246–47; mood changes in, 232–33; older child, 231; reactions to parent's illness, 196; school performance of, 234–35; sleep problems in, 233–34; talking about spirituality with, 196; telling about cancer, 226–32; very young child, 230–31; warning signs that your child needs help, 232–35

chiropractic medicine, 81–82

Chopra, Deepak, 6

Christianity, 204, 206

Christian Scientists, 201

Chronic Pain and the Family (Silver), 156, 219

circadian rhythms, 145, 147

citalopram (Celexa), 186

clinical trials, 60–61, 264, 271

Clinton, Bill, 28, 121

clomipramine (Anafranil), 186

cluster symptoms, 139

Coach Yourself to Success (Miedaner), 42

codeine, 158

cognitive behavioral therapy, 152, 154, 188

Cohn, Ken, 244–45, 249

cold packs for pain, 167–68

colorectal cancer, 24, 95, 98–99, 134, 204

complementary and alternative medicine (CAM), 6, 59; acupuncture, 71–74, 78, 85, 87–89, 90, 172, 192; Ayurvedic medicine, 6, 76, 78–79; botanicals and dietary supplements, 80–81 (*see also* dietary supplements); cancer and, 84–85; combined with conventional medicine, 63, 70–71, 90–91 (*see also* integrative medicine); vs. conventional medicine, 60–63; definition of, 62–63, 70, 71, 75; energy therapies, 76, 83–84; healing and, 87–91; health food store recommendations for, 89–90; herbal remedies, 75–76, 78, 79, 80–81, 86, 87, 89, 275; homeopathy, 77–78, 88; legitimating, 74–76; manipulative and body-based methods, 81–83; mind-body therapies, 79–80, 85, 172, 207; for pain, 70, 71, 72–73, 82, 83, 85, 87–89, 90, 172–73, 207; percentage of persons using, 74–75, 84; quackery, 59, 71, 73, 85–87; reasons for use of, 72; resources for, 90–91, 274–77; spirituality and, 74, 83, 84, 88; traditional Chinese medicine, 78; types of, 76; understanding, 71–74

Complete Guide to Complementary and Alternative Cancer Therapies, 90–91

Consortium of Academic Health Centers for Integrative Medicine, 274

constipation, 127, 137, 138, 159, 164

conventional medicine, 59–60, 63–64; choosing right treatment for you, 66–68; vs. nonconventional, 60–63

cooking/meal preparation, 41–42, 49, 54–55, 147, 231

coping, 31, 176, 181, 190; by children, 226, 232; with pain, 171; religion and, 198, 200

corticosteroids, 146, 161, 168

cortisol, 82, 199

Council of State Administrators of Vocational Rehabilitation, 269

couples and intimacy, 214, 215, 218–26

crisis phase, 31–32, 202–4

Crivello, Madeline, 9, 10

Crusade (Ross), 16

cure, 5, 10, 174, 229; for advanced cancers, 256; alternative therapies and, 70, 72, 77, 84, 86, 87, 89, 90; search for, 252–57; surgical, 19, 253

Curie, Marie, 253

cycling, 106, 107, 108, 113

Cymbalta (duloxetine), 186

dairy products, 122, 130

dancing, 102, 106, 107

A Darker Ribbon (Leopold), 216

Das, Surya, 212

deconditioning, 50, 115

definition of cancer, 17

Deng, Gary, 70–71

denosumab, 160

depression, 65, 68, 176, 178–79, 185, 188–89, 249; alcohol and, 136, 187; CAM therapies for, 87, 167; in children, 234; at end of treatment, 184; exercise for, 94, 97; fatigue and, 140, 141, 142, 143, 153, 154; grief and, 179–80; insomnia and, 146, 147; intimacy and, 219–20, 221; journaling for, 193–94; loneliness and, 239; medications for, 171, 185–87, 188, 190, 191, 194, 221; physical changes causing, 185, 188; in PTSD, 191; recovery and, 27, 28, 182–83; sleep and, 146, 147, 149, 188; social support and, 192, 214; spirituality and, 198, 199, 200; support groups and, 237; symptoms of, 180, 183; talking to doctor about, 187, 189

desipramine (Norpramin), 186

Desyrel (trazodone), 186

diabetes, 102, 113, 129, 143, 201

diagnosis of cancer, 1, 242–43; crisis of, 31–32, 202–4; early detection, 257; telling children about, 226–32; what to do after, 2

diarrhea, 77, 138, 141, 160

diet, 8, 10, 26–27, 118–38, 260; alcohol

exercise (*cont.*)
107, 108, 115, 116, 153–54; fitness and, 94, 97, 99, 103, 109, 114, 115, 142, 153; FITT principle for, 99–100, 103; for flexibility, 50, 96, 99, 110–11, 113, 167; frequency and duration of, 103, 107–8; getting started with, 103–5; isometric, 113; for lumbar stabilization, 113; for mood symptoms, 94, 95, 97, 191–92; pain and, 32, 97, 102, 109, 110–11, 113, 115, 116, 165–67; vs. physical activity, 50; prehabilitation, 21–22; prescription of, 100; to prevent cancer recurrence, 10, 61–62, 94, 95, 117, 257; to rebuild strength and endurance, 25, 50, 53, 96, 97, 99, 104, 106, 107, 108–10, 115, 153; vs. rehabilitation, 12, 13; resistance (strength training), 50, 99, 108–10, 113, 115, 248; specific problems affecting, 112–17; target heart rate for, 104; temperature for, 53; weight-bearing, 113, 128; when to avoid, 113, 116. *See also* physical therapy
exercise testing, 100–102
exhaustion, 3, 9, 42, 52, 53, 140, 142, 148, 247–48. *See also* fatigue

facet blocks, 166
faith, 197, 202, 204, 205–6. *See also* religion; spirituality
The Faith Healers (Randi), 201
faith healing, 201–2
falls, 47, 116, 160
fatigue, 14, 139–55, 247–48; cancer-related, 140–44; causes of, 141–43; chemo brain and, 148–50; depression and, 140, 141, 142, 143, 153, 154; diet for, 136–37, 154; energy conservation/pacing for, 47, 50, 51, 55, 57, 68; evaluation of, 143, 151, 152; exercise for, 94, 95, 96, 97, 107, 108, 115, 116, 153–54; healing and, 140; integrative therapies for, 70, 90; intimacy and, 219, 220; keeping log of, 40, 50, 51; mood and, 182, 183, 189; pain and, 139, 140, 141, 142, 143; sleep and, 139, 144–48, 154; talking to doctor about, 139–40, 151, 153; treatment of, 151–55

fats in diet, 23, 27, 119, 122, 126, 130, 192
fear, 13, 17, 43, 86, 153, 180–81, 182, 193, 242, 244; religious belief and, 198, 208. *See also* anxiety/worry
fertility, 65, 221, 223, 224–26, 273
fiber in diet, 123, 125
fight or flight response, 211
fish, 126, 130
fitness, 94, 97, 99, 109, 115, 142, 153
fitness professionals, 103, 113
flexibility exercises, 50, 96, 99, 110–11, 113, 167
fluoxetine (Prozac), 185, 186
Foley, Brian, 28, 225
food pyramid, 118–19, 129
Ford, Betty, 17
Fox, Michael J., 135
free radicals, 25, 96, 145
French, Marilyn, 3
friendships, 2, 214, 216, 217, 235–37
frozen shoulder, 22, 112
fruits, 23, 27, 48, 121, 122, 123–25, 126, 129, 130, 137, 192
future therapies, 5, 252–58

gabapentin, 158
Gallagher, Hugh Gregory, 48
genetic predisposition, 18
Gilman, Alfred, 5, 253
ginseng, 80
glycemic index, 125
Goals! (Tracy), 32
goals for healing, 33–38, 39, 40, 261; categories of, 37; process of setting, 34; realistic, 35–36; revisiting, 251; setbacks and, 32–33; short- and long-term, 34–35, 37–38; written, 36, 37–38
Goldstein, Michael, 74
Goodman, Louis, 5, 153
grief stages, 179–80, 181, 182
grocery shopping, 37, 41–42, 48, 49, 56–57, 122
Groopman, Jerome, 205
guided imagery, 153, 166, 171, 188
guilt feelings, 28, 35, 62, 103, 132, 175, 180, 181, 183, 232, 235
gynecologic cancers, 199, 252

Hahnemann, Samuel, 77
Harpham, Wendy Schlessel, 226, 227
Harvard School of Public Health, 274
Haynes, Brian, 61
head and neck cancers, 3, 21, 28, 134, 179, 219, 225, 252, 256, 259
Healing Beyond the Body (Dossey), 207
Healing Together (Jampolsky), 27
health food store recommendations, 89–90
health insurance, 66, 266, 281; for rehabilitation, 12, 13, 34; for smoking cessation, 22
heart disease, 65, 143, 169, 177; alcohol and, 134; diet and, 120; exercise and, 93, 97, 99, 102, 117
heart rate, 83, 102, 151, 207, 211; target, for exercise, 104
The Heart's Wisdom: A Practical Guide to Growing through Love (Vissell and Vissell), 224
hepatitis B virus, 256
herbal remedies, 75–76, 78, 79, 80–81, 86, 87, 89, 275. *See also specific herbs*
Herceptin, 245
high-quality care, 13, 64, 66
Hippocrates, 77, 94, 118
Hirschland, Ruth, 94
Hodgkin's lymphoma, 225, 254, 256, 259
holistic medicine, 8, 74, 81, 90
Holland, Jimmie, 176, 178
Holmes, Michelle, 61
homeopathy, 77–78, 88
hope, 2, 27, 31, 179–80, 200, 206, 212, 227, 228, 229, 230, 242, 254
hormones, 66, 83; emotions and, 185, 187, 189; exercise and, 96, 116; fatigue and, 141, 143; in food production, 121, 128, 129; sexuality and, 219, 221; sleep and, 145, 146–47, 152, 188
Horn, John, 75
hot flashes, 85, 87, 148, 152, 153, 185
hot packs for pain, 167–68
household chores, 20, 37, 41–42, 43, 53, 54–56, 147, 169–70
How to Live on 24 Hours a Day (Bennett), 39
How to Pray without Being Religious (Moon), 197

Hoxey, Harry, 86
human immunodeficiency virus (HIV), 256
human papillomavirus (HPV), 252, 256
The Human Side of Cancer: Living with Hope, Coping with Uncertainty (Holland), 176
hydration, 137
hypnosis, 87, 88, 166, 171, 172
hysterectomy, 169, 225, 226

imagery, 88, 150, 190, 192, 210; guided, 153, 166, 171, 188
imaging studies, 2, 31, 257
imipramine (Tofranil), 186
immune function, 25–26, 256; CAM therapies and, 83, 87, 88; cancer recurrence and, 25–26, 167; diet and, 120, 123, 125; exercise and, 96, 97, 108, 109; how to boost, 27; journaling and, 193; massage and, 83, 88, 101, 167; pain and, 163; psychoneuroimmunology, 10, 166–67, 176–77, 198, 199, 202; sleep and, 144–45, 148; spirituality and, 10, 199; stress and, 27, 199, 202; support network and, 214
immune system cells, 25, 199, 202
immunotherapy, 20–21, 115, 256
incontinence, 21, 220
infection, 26, 74, 201; exercise and, 114, 115, 116; fatigue and, 141, 143; HPV, 252, 256; nutritional status and, 120; postoperative, 22, 114, 116, 172; smoking and, 22, 133; treatment-related risk of, 102, 115
infertility, 184, 221, 225–26
inflammation, 23, 96, 166
injections for pain, 165, 166
In Love with Daylight: A Memoir of Recovery (Sheed), 3
insomnia, 143, 144, 146–47, 152. *See also* sleep problems
Institute of Medicine, 65–66, 175–76
insulin, 23, 96, 125, 137
integrative medicine, 63, 70–71, 88, 90–91, 274
intentional healing, 26
The Interactive Healthy Eating Index, 275

interferon, 21, 141, 145

interleukins, 21, 141, 145, 147

Internet information, 16, 72, 119, 246. *See also* resources

interval training, 108, 115

intimacy, 214; cancer factors affecting, 219–20; couples and, 214, 215, 218–26; definition of, 219; emotional, 219, 221, 222; fertility and, 65, 223, 224–26; improving, 221–24; nonsexual, 224; physical, 219, 220–23, 224; talking to doctor about, 223

iontophoresis, 168

iron deficiency, 125, 127, 137, 143

Jampolsky, Lee, 27

Jefferson, Thomas, 201

Jenks, Will, 240

joint injections, 165, 166

Jordan, Hamilton, 174

journaling, 193–94

Judaism, 204, 205, 206, 208

Kaelin, Carolyn, 95, 243–44, 245

Kaposi's sarcoma, 256

Keep It Simple (Bradshaw), 45

Keith, Toby, 261

Keller, Helen, 258

Kicking Butts, 134

kidney cancer, 19, 204, 237

Kids Konnected, 272

kingdom of the sick, 3–6

Koenig, Harold, 197, 199, 202

Kolata, Gina, 94

Kolb, Claudia, 193

Koob, Kathryn, 193

Kraus, Hans, 94

Krieger, Delores, 83

Kübler-Ross, Elisabeth, 179

Kuhlman, Katherine, 201

laboratory reports, 2

Landers, Ann, 133

Lasser, Terese, 238

lateral epicondylitis, 89

laundry/dry cleaning, 49, 50, 53, 55

Leopold, Ellen, 216

leukemia, 204, 219, 253, 255, 264–65

Leukemia and Lymphoma Society, 264–65

Lexapro (escitalopram), 186

libido, decreased, 131, 149, 157, 186, 219, 220, 223

lidocaine, 164

The Link between Religion and Health (Koenig and Cohen), 199

Lipe, Jay, 36

Livestrong Fertility, 273

Livestrong Foundation, 265

Living a Connected Life (Brehony), 239

Living through Breast Cancer (Kaelin), 96, 243

loneliness, 239

Look Good . . . Feel Better, 265

love and healing, 214, 224, 240. *See also* support system

Love and Survival (Ornish), 214

Lucky Man (Fox), 135

lung cancer, 18, 21, 37, 160, 202, 204, 256, 266

lymphedema, 85, 89, 114, 161–62, 171–72, 269

lymphoma, 242, 243, 244, 256, 264–65; Hodgkin's, 225, 254, 256, 259; non-Hodgkin's, 174, 203, 216, 226, 253

manipulative and body-based methods, 81–83

manual therapy, 168–69

massage, therapeutic, 79, 82–83, 85, 88, 101, 192; for pain, 166, 167, 168, 169, 172

mastectomy, 7, 17, 89, 112, 165, 185, 215, 238, 244

McKown v. Lundman, 201

Mead, Margaret, 207

Meals on Wheels Association of America, 275

meat, 119, 122, 126, 128, 130

medical records, 2

meditation, 28, 37, 52, 74, 79, 88, 136, 150, 212; breath-focused, 209; definition of, 79, 207; to improve mood, 188, 190, 192, 207; mindfulness, 207, 209; for pain, 166, 172, 207; prayer and, 197, 206, 207; spirituality and,

207, 209–10; transcendental, 210; visualization and imagery, 210
Meili, Trisha, 14
melanoma, 102, 174, 204
melatonin, 145
Memorial Sloan-Kettering Cancer Center, 275
menopause, treatment-induced, 185, 223, 225
mental health professionals, 188–91
mental health resources, 278–80
metastasis, 18
Miedaner, Talane, 42
mild cognitive impairment (MCI), 148–50
mind-body therapies, 79–80, 85, 172, 207
mindfulness, 30, 207, 209
mirtazapine (Remeron), 186
mood symptoms, 27, 136, 174–95; alcohol use and, 135–36, 187; baseline, 178–82; in children, 232–33; consulting mental health professionals for, 188–91; distress screening, 65–66, 67, 176; exercise for, 94, 95, 97, 191–92; fatigue, sleep, and, 146, 153, 154, 183, 188; intimacy and, 219–20, 221; link between emotional and physical health, 175–78; physical factors affecting, 185–87; quality of life and, 176, 178–79, 183, 187, 191, 192, 250; recovery and, 182–85; stages of grief, 179–80, 181, 182; strategies for improving, 191–95; talking to doctor about, 187–88, 189, 191; working toward emotional balance, 187–88. *See also* anxiety/worry; depression; fear
Moon, Janell, 197, 207
morphine, 158
muscle relaxants, 164, 165, 221
musculoskeletal pain, 71, 102, 157, 163, 165, 172; acupuncture for, 85, 88–89
music, 52, 79, 87, 150, 204
Muslims, 206
mustard gas, 5, 253
My Breast (Wadler), 215
myofascial release techniques, 169

napping, 52, 143, 147, 150, 153, 154, 216, 248
Nash, Jennie, 215
National Association of Social Workers, 279–80
National Cancer Institute, 131, 254, 265
National Center for Complementary and Alternative Medicine (NCCAM), 62–63, 75, 76, 131, 275
National Coalition for Cancer Survivorship, 265
National Comprehensive Cancer Network, 140, 266
National Heart, Lung, and Blood Institute Health Information Center, 275
National Institutes of Health (NIH), 61, 62, 72, 75
National Library of Medicine, 266
National Lymphedema Network, 269
National Osteoporosis Foundation, 127
Native American medicine men, 206
nausea/vomiting, 116, 138, 141, 174; CAM therapies for, 72, 85, 87, 89; cannabinoids for, 161; drug-induced, 159, 164, 186
NeedyMeds, 280–81
nefazodone (Serzone), 186
nerve blocks, 165, 166
neuropathy, 7, 134–35, 163–64
neurotransmitters, 185, 186, 187
New Age medicine, 90
"new normal," 14, 33, 44
nicotine/tobacco use, 18, 22, 24, 75, 77, 130, 132–34, 150, 181, 198, 200, 257; quitting smoking, 22, 133–34, 186
Nixon, Richard, 72
Nolen, William, 201
nonconventional medicine, 60–63; combined with conventional medicine, 63, 70–71, 90–91, 274. *See also* complementary and alternative medicine; integrative medicine
nonsteroidal anti-inflammatory drugs (NSAIDs), 164
norepinephrine, 144, 185, 186
Norpramin (desipramine), 186
nortriptyline (Pamelor), 186
No Such Thing as a Bad Day (Jordan), 174

obesity/overweight, 23, 96, 98, 105, 119, 149
occupational therapists, 40, 50, 167, 168, 268
occupational therapy, 12, 34, 102, 115, 165
Office for the Study of Unconventional Medical Practices, 75
oils in diet, 126, 130
Olson, James, 59, 86, 254
opioids for pain, 142, 157–60, 164, 165; potential problems with, 158; signs of withdrawal or intoxication with, 160
optimal healing, 10, 14, 26, 30, 50, 119, 183, 250
optimism, 6, 33, 66, 97, 178, 200, 248, 254
organic foods, 48, 122, 128–29, 130
Ornish, Dean, 214, 240
osteopathy, 81, 82
osteopenia/osteoporosis, 82, 83, 88, 113, 127–28
ostomy, exercise and, 114
O'Terry, Candy, 9
ovarian cancer, 204, 219, 260, 266
overwhelmed feelings, 38–39, 79, 121, 140, 143, 185, 193, 238, 247

pacing, 26, 44, 48–58, 154; basics of, 51–53; tips for, 54–58
pain, 1, 14, 46, 65, 115, 139, 156–63, 259; back, 45, 73, 90, 97, 110–11, 113, 161–62, 163, 165, 169; bone, 160–61; exercise and, 32, 97, 102, 109, 110–11, 113, 115, 116; fatigue and, 139, 140, 141, 142, 143; fear of, 180; fine-tuning your pain filter, 162–63; intimacy and, 219–20, 223; malignant, 157–61; mood and, 183; musculoskeletal, 71, 85, 88–89, 102, 157, 163, 165, 172; neuropathic, 7, 134–35, 163–64; nociceptive, 163, 164; nonmalignant, 161–62; pacing and, 53; shoulder, 7, 22, 112, 139, 185; sleep and, 146, 148, 152, 153, 187, 188; after surgery, 3, 89, 112, 115, 146; talking to doctor about, 250; three-day log of, 40, 50, 51; as vital sign, 156
pain management, 8, 27, 68, 163–73, 260; CAM therapies for, 70, 71, 72–73, 82, 83, 85, 87–89, 90, 172–73,
207; equipment for, 169; exercise for, 165–67; lifestyle changes for, 169–71; other modalities for, 167–69; psychological intervention for, 171; resources for, 277–78; spirituality and, 200, 203–4, 208; surgery for, 171–72
pain medications, 68, 146; anti-inflammatory drugs, 158, 164, 165; injections, 165, 166; ladder approach to, 158; for malignant pain, 157–61; for nonmalignant pain, 163–65, 166; opioids, 142, 157–60, 164, 165; topical, 163, 164–65
Pamelor (nortriptyline), 186
pancreatic cancer, 134
parenting. See children of cancer patient
paroxetine (Paxil), 185, 186
Partnership for Prescription Assistance, 281
Paxil (paroxetine), 185, 186
pedometer, 2, 105–6
pelvic floor exercises, 21
Pennebaker, James, 193–94
Pennsylvania Dutch, 206
pessimism, 177, 178
Petri, Anette Lykke, 135
physiatrists, 4, 67, 68, 100, 157, 190, 267. See also rehabilitation specialists
physical activity, 2, 8; vs. exercise, 50; pacing for, 48–58; after surgery, 20; three-day log of, 40–41, 42, 50–51
physical healing, 5, 6–8, 11, 16–28; CAM therapies and, 87–91; diet and, 120, 122, 123, 124, 129–31; emotional healing and, 26, 32, 37; fatigue and, 140; finding time for, 38–43; focusing on, 31–32; how we heal best, 26–28; immune system and, 25–26; optimal, 10, 14, 26, 30, 50, 119, 183, 250; plateaus during, 247–48; setbacks during, 27, 32–33, 35, 183, 243–47, 260; setting goals for, 32–38, 251, 261; striving for progress in, 248–51
physical therapists, 64, 100, 103, 112, 114, 168, 268
physical therapy, 12, 34, 100, 112, 165, 168, 192; prescription for, 99, 100, 112; safe and unsafe techniques, 100, 101

phytochemicals, 123–24, 125, 131
plateaus during recovery, 247–48
Popoff, Peter, 201–2
posttraumatic growth, 202–3
posttraumatic stress disorder (PTSD), 184, 191
Potter, Jennifer, 219
prayer, 10, 28, 52, 79–80, 88, 134, 192, 196, 197, 203–7, 211, 212; definition of, 197; faith healing, 201–2; for healing, 208; intercessory, 205; meditation and, 197, 206, 207. *See also* religion; spirituality
Prayer Is Good Medicine (Dossey), 205
precision medicine, 257
prehabilitation, 2, 6, 7, 11, 21–25, 33, 98–99, 120, 192, 243, 250, 260
prevention of cancer, 5, 10, 19, 145, 252; diet for, 120, 124, 257; exercise for, 93, 94–95, 117, 257; melatonin for, 145; primary, 257; secondary, 257; vaccines for, 5, 21, 252, 256
prioritizing, 40, 43, 44, 45–48; goal setting and, 35, 38; pacing and, 49, 50
problem-oriented care, 7
prognosis, 2, 9, 24, 72, 96, 140, 177, 180–81, 190, 228, 231, 237–38, 243–47, 256
prostate cancer, 21, 24, 37, 152, 157, 160, 174, 199, 204, 219, 266
protein in diet, 120, 121, 122, 123, 130, 136; supplementation of, 22, 98, 120, 122
Prozac (fluoxetine), 185, 186
psychiatrists, 171, 179, 189, 190, 224, 227
psychological interventions, 188–91; for children of cancer patient, 232–35; for pain, 171. *See also* mood symptoms
psychologists, 64, 171, 189, 190, 197, 224, 230, 268, 270, 279
psychoneuroimmunology, 10, 166–67, 176–77, 198, 199, 202
psychostimulants, 152
Putnam, Robert, 239

quackery, 59, 71, 73, 85–87
Quackwatch, Inc., 276
quality of life, 8, 49, 50; exercise and, 94, 95, 96, 97; fatigue and, 139, 151; mood and, 176, 178–79, 183, 187, 191,

192, 250; spirituality and, 10, 198–99; support system and, 192, 214, 235, 237
quitting smoking, 22, 133–34, 186

radiation therapy, 3, 5, 19, 21, 66, 85, 96, 184, 254; exercise and, 102, 112, 115; fatigue due to, 141–42; herbal remedies and, 81; history of, 253; secondary malignancies and, 259; spirituality and, 199; after surgery, 20
radiopharmaceuticals, 161
Raising an Emotionally Healthy Child When a Parent Is Sick (Rauch), 227
Randi, James, 201
Rauch, Paula, 227–28
Reach for Recovery, 238
recurrence of cancer, 32, 59, 161, 244, 247; diet and, 123, 257; energetics to decrease risk of, 24, 257; exercise and, 10, 61–62, 94, 95, 117, 257; HER-2 positive breast cancer, 245; immune function and, 25–26, 167; monitoring for, 250; mood and, 136, 178, 183, 184; prevention of, 10, 19, 89, 257
rehabilitation, 7, 44, 100, 190, 192; asking doctor about, 2, 243, 250, 260; dual screening for, 66, 67, 176; vs. exercise and wellness services, 12, 13; health insurance for, 12, 13, 34; impairment-driven, 13; prehabilitation and, 99, 243; religiousness and, 198; resources for, 267–70; setting goals for, 33–34, 36–37; sexual, 223–24; STAR Program, 11–12, 13, 67, 269–70; vocational, 269
Rehabilitation of Sports Injuries (Audette), 88
rehabilitation specialists, 4, 8, 10, 12, 33, 34, 39, 67–68, 94, 100, 103, 113, 173, 190, 192, 243, 259, 268
Reiki, 83
Reiter, Russel, 145
rejection feelings, 217, 239
relaxation, 49, 52, 150
The Relaxation Response (Benson), 211
relaxation techniques, 74, 79, 82, 87–88, 150, 153, 190, 192, 209; for pain, 166

religion, 27, 83–84, 122, 129, 136, 196–207, 216; definition of, 197; fraud, faith healing, and, 201–2; health and, 198–200; prayer and, 205–8. *See also* prayer; spirituality

Remeron (mirtazapine), 186

remission, 5, 142

reproductive health, 272; fertility, 65, 221, 223, 224–26, 273

resistance exercises, 50, 99, 108–10, 113, 115, 248

resources, 42, 263–81

rest, 26–27, 37, 49, 50, 52–53, 108, 143, 150, 154, 192, 260; naps, 52, 143, 147, 150, 153, 154, 216, 248. *See also* sleep

Ritalin, 152

Rodgers, Joni, 216

role changes, 4, 38, 219

Rollin, Betty, 17

Ross, Walter, 16

Saper, Robert, 76

scarring, 20; exercise and, 102, 112, 115; pain from, 115, 157, 162

Schilling, Curt, 63

Schneider, Myra, 193

Schneiderman, Eric, 80

Schnipper, Hester Hill, 227

school performance of children, 234–35

Schover, Leslie, 224

screening tests, 5; for cancer survivors, 65–66; dual screening, 66, 67, 176; in fatigue workup, 152

Sealy, Patricia, 203

A Season in Hell (French), 3

second opinion, 2, 24, 31, 169

selective serotonin reuptake inhibitors (SSRIs), 185, 186

self-esteem, 192, 200, 239

sentinel symptoms, 139

serotonin, 160, 185, 186

serotonin norepinephrine reuptake inhibitors (SNRIs), 185, 186

sertraline (Zoloft), 185, 186

Serzone (nefazodone), 186

setbacks during recovery, 27, 32–33, 35, 183, 243–47, 260

sex therapy, 224

sexual dysfunction clinics, 224

sexuality, 219–24, 270; decreased libido, 131, 149, 157, 186, 219, 220, 223; drugs affecting, 186, 220, 221; pain and, 219–20, 223

Sexuality and Infertility after Cancer (Schover), 224

sexual rehabilitation, 223–24

shame, 16, 216, 225

SHARE (Self-Help for Women with Breast or Ovarian Cancer), 266

Sharing Good Times (Carter), 218

Sheed, Wilfred, 3

shoulder: acupuncture for injuries of, 88; breast cancer–related symptoms in, 7, 22, 112, 139, 185; injections for bursitis in, 166

Sinequan (doxepin), 186

6-minute walk (run) test, 105

skin cancer, 102, 127, 174, 204, 255

skin changes, 18; on breast, 244; drug-induced, 164; exercise and, 115

sleep, 2, 8, 26–27; duration of, 148; keeping log of, 154; stages of, 146

sleep apnea, 143, 147, 148, 149

sleep hygiene, 148, 150, 152

sleep problems, 7; in children, 233–34; fatigue due to, 139, 144–48, 154; grief and, 180; immune function and, 144–45, 148; insomnia, 143, 144, 146–47, 152; mood and, 183; pain and, 146, 148, 152, 153, 187, 188. *See also* rest

smoking cessation, 22, 133–34, 186. *See also* nicotine/tobacco use

social capital, 238–40

Social Security Disability Insurance, 267

social withdrawal/alienation, 216, 239

social workers, 171, 189, 190, 224, 227, 270, 279

Somers, Suzanne, 66

Sontag, Susan, 3

soy, 131–32

speech therapy, 12, 34, 268, 269

spirituality, 10, 196–212, 260, 279; CAM therapies and, 74, 83, 84, 88; definition of, 197; doing what works for you, 212; healing and, 27, 28; health and, 198–200; immune function and, 10, 199; meditation, 207, 209–10;

treatments for cancer (*cont.*)
quackery, 59, 71, 73, 85–87; radiation therapy, 19, 21; surgery, 19–20; survivorship as component of, 64–66; targeted therapy, 5, 19, 20, 21, 256–57; toxicity of, 1–5
trigger-point injections, 165, 166
triggers and tendencies for cancer, 18–19
Twain, Mark, 106

Ultimate Fitness (Kolata), 94
ultrasound, 31, 177; therapeutic, 101, 167, 168
underweight, 23, 105, 126
U.S. Department of Agriculture (USDA), 118–19, 128–29; Food and Nutrition Information Center, 276
U.S. Food and Drug Administration (FDA), 60, 76, 80–81, 86, 277
uterine cancer, 96, 152, 161, 184, 204, 219, 225

vaccines, 5, 20–21, 252, 254, 256
vegetables, 23, 27, 48, 121, 122, 123–25, 126, 129, 130, 137, 192
venlafaxine (Effexor), 185, 186
The Victoria's Secret Catalog Never Stops Coming (Nash), 215
viruses and cancer, 256
Vissell, Barry, 224
Vissell, Joyce, 224
visualization, 210
vitamin B complex, 125
vitamin C, 123
vitamin D, 127–28, 130
vitamin E, 123, 125
vitamins/minerals: in diet, 120, 121, 123; megadoses of, 73, 88, 89, 124–25; supplements of, 22, 80, 124–25, 127–28, 130
vocational rehabilitation, 269

Wadler, Joyce, 215
walking, 7, 21, 23, 45, 46–47, 50, 94, 102, 103, 106, 107, 134, 167, 222, 226; energy conservation and, 54, 57; fatigue and, 108, 244; setting goals for, 35, 37; 6-minute walk test, 105
Watkins, Shirley, 119
weight, 22–23, 98, 105, 120, 122, 142, 276; BMI and, 105; depression and, 183; diet, exercise, and, 22–24, 98–99; diet and, 126, 129, 137, 138, 234; drug-induced changes in, 164, 186; intimacy and, 219, 220
weight-bearing exercise, 113, 128
weight lifting, 109–10, 114, 248
Weihs, Karen, 214
Wellbutrin (bupropion), 186
The Well Spouse Association, 273
What Helped Get Me Through: Cancer Survivors Share Wisdom and Hope (Silver), 2, 203
When a Parent Has Cancer (Harpham), 226
When God and Cancer Meet (Eib), 212
whole grains, 122, 125, 126, 130
Willett, Walter, 118–19, 120
worry. *See* anxiety/worry
Writing My Way through Cancer (Schneider), 193
Writing to Heal (Pennebaker), 193

yard work, 42, 49, 50, 56
yoga, 79, 88, 102, 111, 212
Young Survival Coalition, 267
You've Got a Friend (Zadra), 237

Zoloft (sertraline), 185, 186